# Social Media in Healthcare:
## Connect, Communicate, Collaborate

---

Your board, staff, or clients may also benefit from this book's insight. For more information on quantity discounts, contact the Health Administration Press Marketing Manager at (312) 424-9470.

This publication is intended to provide accurate and authoritative information in regard to the subject matter covered. It is sold, or otherwise provided, with the understanding that the publisher is not engaged in rendering professional services. If professional advice or other expert assistance is required, the services of a competent professional should be sought.

The statements and opinions contained in this book are strictly those of the author and do not represent the official positions of the American College of Healthcare Executives or the Foundation of the American College of Healthcare Executives.



15 14 13 12 11 5 4 3

**Library of Congress Cataloging-in-Publication Data**

Thielst, Christina Beach.
Social media in healthcare : connect, communicate, collaborate / Christina Thielst.
p. cm.
ISBN 978-1-56793-356-7
1. Social media. 2. Medical informatics. I. Title.
R859.T55 2010
610.285–dc22
2009050525

The paper used in this publication meets the minimum requirements of American National Standard for Information Sciences—Permanence of Paper for Printed Library Materials, ANSI Z39.48-1984. ♾™

Acquisitions editor: Eileen Lynch; Project manager: Dojna Shearer; Cover designer: Scott Miller; Layout: BookComp

Found an error or a typo? We want to know!
Please e-mail it to hap1@ache.org, and put "Book Error" in the subject line.

For photocopying and copyright information, please contact Copyright Clearance Center at www.copyright.com or at (978) 750-8400.

Health Administration Press
A division of the Foundation of the American
College of Healthcare Executives
One North Franklin Street, Suite 1700
Chicago, IL 60606-3529
(312) 424-2800

CHAPTER 1

# Starting a Conversation

**Social media** are electronic tools that enhance communication, support collaboration, and enable users across the globe to generate and share content. The various forms of social media allow users to build social networks and start conversations with those who share their interests and experiences. The subjects of these conversations range from pure entertainment to harnessing the collective knowledge needed to answer life's most pressing questions. The result is unlike more traditional media vehicles—such as TV, radio, newspapers, and **websites**—that typically only push out information after it has been scripted, edited, produced, and staged. ▶

**Social media**—online content created by people using highly accessible and scalable publishing technologies. In its most basic sense, social media represents a shift in how people discover, read, and share news, information, and content. It fuses sociology and technology, transforming monologues (a communication from one to many) into dialogues (two-way communication) and democratizes information, transforming content readers into publishers. Social media is popular because it allows people to form online relationships for personal, political, and business use. Businesses also refer to social media as user-generated content (UGC) or consumer-generated media (CGM).

**Website**—A collection of related Web pages, images, videos, or other digital assets that are addressed with a common domain name or Internet protocol (IP) address in an IP-based network. A website is hosted on at least one Web server, accessible via the Internet or a private local area network.

---

Social media and its networking capabilities originated with the launch of Friendster (www.friendster.com), the first online social network. A privately owned website, Friendster focused on helping people meet new friends and stay in touch with old ones through sharing online content and media. Since 2002, the reasons for forming and joining social networks have matured, and now they are limited only by our imaginations. Over the last several years, the growth of social networking options has been dramatic, and the various applications are quickly finding their way into business and health organizations around the world.

This book provides an overview of various social media tools and examples of how they are used in healthcare and community health environments to connect with the public, employees, physicians, consumers, and other stakeholders. It will stimulate readers to consider new uses for media in the healthcare environment and in their organizations. I hope that by the time each reader reaches the end of the book, he or she will be able to identify a tool that can improve outreach into a particular community, whether it is

- internal to the organization;
- geographically isolated, rural, surburban, or urban;
- disease- or condition-specific;
- demographically oriented; or
- widespread—*the masses*.

Each chapter of this book defines and describes a social media tool and reviews its costs, benefits, sample uses, and any limitations and risks specific to healthcare environments. We will explore the language of social media and its value proposition for the healthcare industry and encourage readers to explore the many sites and materials referenced.

## OUR COMMUNITY AND PATIENTS

Healthcare is undergoing an unprecedented transformation. Cost, quality, safety, and staffing challenges are giving rise to a new, more proactive role for the average patient.

Social media provide people with additional opportunities to enhance their knowledge and their ability to care for themselves, and online communities are attracting older and broader audiences. For some, social networks are just new information and communication tools that are becoming as much a part of their daily lives as newspapers, radio, TV, and the telephone. In fact, producers of traditional media have already recognized this fundamental shift in where people go for information, and they too are applying social media tools to broaden their outreach, audience, and attractiveness.

## OUR WORKFORCE AND OTHER STAKEHOLDERS

Healthcare leaders are expected to improve quality, safety, and productivity, often at the same time they are being asked to decrease costs. Successful leaders understand the importance of communication and collaboration during challenging times and seek tools that allow them to reach out to physicians, employees, volunteers, and others more effectively and efficiently.

Proactive leaders are exploring the low-cost—but potentially high-touch—social media applications and incorporating those that fit into their strategic initiatives. Correctly applied, these tools can improve the quality of information and the efficiency at which it is gathered, shared, and used. These new tools help healthcare leaders listen, learn, and build on their organization's collective knowledge with new relationships and increased trust.

## WEB 1.0

In the early 1990s, the Internet and websites were new, and each had recognizable and unknown potential. Traditional read-only websites (**Web 1.0**) provide access to the information a healthcare organization believes its stakeholders need, and the information remains the same until the organization replaces it with something it believes to be more valuable. And, once a stakeholder locates needed information, he or she can only access it as long as the organization keeps it on the site. To many, these first generation websites seem static or stale unless they are frequently updated with content that accurately reflects stakeholder needs and expectations.

---

**Web 1.0**—A retronym that refers to the state of the World Wide Web and any website design style used before the advent of Web 2.0; a general term created to describe the Web before the bursting of the dot-com bubble in 2001, which was a turning point for the Internet.

---

For the purposes of this book, a healthcare organization's stakeholders and potential social media audiences include

- patients, their families, and their friends;
- medical staff and other physicians and allied providers;
- employees and potential employees;
- consumers;
- employers;
- volunteers and auxiliary members;
- grant makers and donors;
- vendors and other partners;
- health plans and payers;
- nonacute care and other support providers;
- media;
- the community at large; and
- licensing, regulatory, and accrediting organizations.

## WEB 2.0, HEALTH 2.0

The idea of **Web 2.0** involves the transformation of relationships by delivering what customers want—personalized information, convenience, and tools to help them plan and execute 24 hours a day, 7 days a week. Social media complement and go beyond the traditional website by actively engaging individuals in their search for information and knowledge and offering an open venue for discussions and user contributions. They

- introduce at least bidirectional capability,
- provide an avenue for dialogue and collaboration in building the content,
- offer easier downloading of content into an individual's personal

collection so that the content is available for as long as he or she wants it,

- allow interested individuals to invite your content into their lives as they want to receive it,
- facilitate the widespread sharing of messages and calls to action, and
- provide access to information while users are at home, at work or school, or mobile.

---

**Web 2.0**—A second generation of Web development and Web design. It facilitates communication, information sharing, interoperability, user-centered design, and collaboration on the World Wide Web. It has led to the development and evolution of Web-based communities, hosted services, and Web applications. Examples include social-networking sites, video-sharing sites, wikis, blogs, mashups, and folksonomies.

---

Unlike Web 1.0, Web 2.0 is created and shaped by the healthcare organization *and* by its users, and it has the potential to evolve with every interaction. Users promote content each time they include a link on a **blog** or other social networking post, and this increases the potential for viral or mass distribution and for mainstream media to pick up on even the most obscure post.

---

**Blog**—A contraction of the term *weblog*; a type of website, usually maintained by an individual with regular entries consisting of commentary, descriptions of events, or other material such as graphics or video. Entries are commonly displayed in reverse-chronological order.

---

*In today's competitive environment, it isn't enough just to have a Web presence. Instead, healthcare organizations need to have* online visibility.

In today's competitive environment, it isn't enough just to have a Web presence. Instead, healthcare organizations need *online visibility,* which is greatly aided by social media content that increases your search engine rating and moves your site toward the first page.

Web 2.0 has led to **Health 2.0**, which, in addition to social media, includes telemedicine, electronic health records, personal health records, and home monitoring. It centers on the idea that patients prefer to take a more active role in gathering and sharing their health information. Tom Ferguson, MD (2007), shares this view of patients being more actively involved:

> [B]ringing healthcare into the new century will not be merely a matter of automating or upgrading our existing clinical processes. We can't just automate earlier forms of medical practice. The underlying nature of healthcare itself must change.

---

**Health 2.0**—Healthcare characterized by the ability to rapidly share, classify, and summarize individual health information with the goals of improving healthcare systems, experiences, and outcomes. Health 2.0 refers to a number of related concepts including telemedicine, electronic medical records, and the use of the Internet by patients through message boards, blogs, and other systems. A key concept is that patients themselves have greater insight into and control of information generated about them.

---

One important agent of this change is e-patients, whom Ferguson defines as

> citizens with health concerns who use the Internet as a health resource, studying up on their own diseases (and those of friends and family members), finding better treatment centers and insisting on better care, providing other patients with invaluable medical assistance and support and increasingly serving as important collaborators and advisors for their clinicians.

These e-patients are becoming more engaged with those who offer opportunities for active participation. They promote the sites and services that best fill their unique disease- or condition-specific needs, such as those that provide virtual support for chronic conditions and information on diagnoses or medications. Patients who are actively engaged often remain on these sites longer, return more often, and share their experiences with others, who in turn pass those stories along to their family and friends.

In addition to their value to patients and the community, social media and networking tools are used in the workplace for administrative and operational purposes. A blog might serve as a suggestion box, providing a forum for employees and patients to share feedback and giving you an opportunity to offer real-time but thoughtful responses. And a wiki may help a multidisciplinary workgroup pull together data and information needed for a report, proposal, application, or plan.

Collaboration is common in healthcare, especially when leaders believe in the collective knowledge of their management team and the value of multidisciplinary approaches to challenges. Social media facilitate this collaboration by bringing people together, providing a forum for questions, collecting answers and ideas, bringing information to the surface, and gathering feedback on interim deliverables.

Social media tools can enhance the gathering of knowledge by allowing wider participation in and contribution to discussions and decisions. Tremendous value can result when a project team uses social media to facilitate and document intelligence gathering or brainstorming sessions, protocol and procedure development, survey preparations, and strategic planning.

Your staff may already be using social media tools for collaboration and communication with partner or professional organizations. Their knowledge of the various tools and their ability to navigate social networking sites will prove valuable to your organization as it evaluates and plans for the application of these new technologies with your key stakeholder groups.

## BOOK COMPANION

A book companion website is available at www.ache.org/books/social. The site includes examples of best practices from healthcare organizations that have successfully begun using social media tools and a list of links to resources for readers who would like additional information.

CHAPTER 2

# The Stats

Healthcare leaders often base decisions on data, which has led to the increasing use of such terms as "evidence-based medicine," "best practices," and "benchmarking" in the workplace. While many healthcare organizations are just starting to track performance indicators related to social media, the explosive growth of e-media has generated statistics that are worth noting.

In 2009, two-thirds of the world's Internet population visited a social networking or blogging site, and this activity accounted for almost 10 percent of all Internet time (Nielsen 2009a). According to Oneupweb (2009b), there were 94.1 million blog readers and 55 million Facebook users in 2008 in the United States alone, and LinkedIn grew 117 percent, from 2.9 million in 2007 to 6.3 million in 2008. The use of these and other social media tools and the relevance of their content have been noted by the search engines, which now ▶

include social media sites on the first page of results.

## HEALTHCARE CONSUMERS USE SOCIAL MEDIA

Consumers are going online to find and share information about topics that affect their healthcare choices, and 34 percent of health searchers use social media resources to delve into health and wellness topics. More men than women appear to use social media to research health and wellness issues (iCrossing 2008). More than 50 percent of adult Internet users in the United States are using social media to find a doctor to treat a specific condition, research the reputation/quality of a doctor or healthcare facility, find out more about the cost of medical procedures/equipment, or access/manage personal health records, and 75 percent are connecting with other consumers to exchange information or get support (iCrossing 2008).

The PEW Research Center reports that 61 percent of U.S. adults look online for health information (Fox and Jones 2009). Of those, 59 percent have also read someone else's commentary; consulted rankings or reviews of doctors, hospitals, or other medical facilities; signed up to receive updates about health or medical issues; or listened to a **podcast** about health or medical issues. In addition, 20 percent of Internet users who have looked online for health information have actively contributed comments, reviews, and updates. In sum, 60 percent of these e-patients (37 percent of U.S. adults) use the interactive features as a supplement to traditional information sources and to deepen their understanding of a condition and sharpen their questions for health professionals.

*The use of these and other social media tools and the relevance of content have been noted by the search engines, which now include social media sites on the first page of results.*

---

**Podcast**—A blend of the words "iPod" and "broadcast." A podcast is a series of digital computer files, usually either audio or video, released periodically and made available for download by means of Web syndication. Like the term "broadcast," podcast can refer to the content itself or to the method by which that content is syndicated; the latter is also called *podcasting*. A podcaster is the person who creates the content.

---

The report concluded that while U.S. adults continue to consult traditional sources of information, such as health professionals, trusted friends, or wise family members, they also go online to obtain information on hospitals or other medical facilities (28%), doctors or other health professionals (35%), and health insurance (27%) (Fox and Jones 2009).

*While American adults continue to consult traditional sources of information, such as health professionals, trusted friends, or wise family members, they also go online to obtain information on hospitals or other medical facilities, doctors or other health professionals, and health insurance.*

Already, 78 percent of baby boomers use the Web to gather health information, and nearly 80 percent of healthcare consumers are interested in accessing their medical records and test results online, scheduling visits online, and connecting with their providers online. The baby boom generation, because of its sheer size and rates of chronic illness, has a greater need than any other generation for interactive online tools for healthcare (Kemper and Mettler 2008), and its members are likely to be the ones driving further growth.

Consumers are also going online for information and assistance as they assume more responsibility for the payment of their healthcare services. As U.S. unemployment hovers around 10 percent, visits to major health insurance providers' websites have declined, but interactive sites offering resources to assist with insurance options have seen increases of 10 to 254 percent as Americans without healthcare coverage or with inadequate coverage explore their options (Comscore 2009).

U.S. Bank (2008) has recognized this need for decision-making support for those paying a greater share of their healthcare costs and is partnering with WebMD to offer enhanced online health tools to its Health Savings Account (HSA) customers. These tools include medication and hospital comparison tools, healthcare calculators, and information guides.

The relationship between online healthcare information seekers and their physicians continues to evolve from a one-way doctor-to-patient lecture into a conversation. A study focusing on technology trends among U.S. physicians found that almost all physicians report that at least some of their patients bring health information they found on the Internet to their appointments, and most of these physicians report spending more time with these patients as a result (Manhattan Research 2009).

## PHYSICIANS AND OTHER STAFF USE SOCIAL MEDIA

Physicians are adopting new media sources, such as online video, podcasts, and blogs, at higher rates than the average consumer. The average physician is more likely to own an iPod than the average 18- to 34-year-old male. Sixty-four percent of U.S. physicians report that they own a PDA or smartphone, and more than half view them as essential tools in their professional practices. The growing number of content providers offering medical information in a variety of formats is expected to increase new media consumption among physicians (Manhattan Research 2009).

Social networking isn't just for patients and physicians. Companies are incorporating these tools into their intranets and allowing employees to use external collaboration sites to increase their productivity and efficiency. Employers are also offering their employees health and wellness programs, which usually include interactive social networking components for support and monitoring progress. According to a study of manufacturers (Capps and Barkley 2008), 77 percent of employers offer formal health and wellness programs, and more than half of those who don't plan to add them. Of those measuring return on investment (ROI), 83 percent estimate it will be greater than break-even.

## HOSPITALS USE SOCIAL MEDIA

And finally, as of this writing, 540 hospitals are using a variety of social media tools (Bennet 2009), including

- 247 YouTube channels,
- 316 Facebook pages,
- 419 Twitter accounts, and
- 67 blogs.

CHAPTER 3

# Overcoming Barriers and Risks

Most people involved with social networking recognize the inherent risks. They simply feel that the value of being part of the conversation and of having readily available avenues to respond to concerns and misunderstandings outweighs the risks. Losses are controlled with few or no adverse effects when organizations are engaged with social media and can quickly identify demoralized employees, dissatisfied consumers or patients, frustrated visitors, and misinformation.

## BE AWARE OF THE CONVERSATION

Today's healthcare leaders need to know what is being said on social networking sites about their organizations, and they need to be prepared to join the conversation to agree, disagree, or offer additional information. In addition ▶

to the organizations represented in the online book companion, health insurers have recognized the risk of not being a part of the conversation and are actively moving to monitor comments being made on blogs, microblogs, and other social networking sites (Mathews 2009).

Your patients, employees, physicians, and other stakeholders are already using Twitter (a microblog), writing or commenting on blog posts, and participating in social networking sites. Mayo Clinic, for example, estimates that more than 5,000 of its employees already use Facebook and recognizes that any one of them can post a comment on a blog or send out a tweet. And when Akron Children's Hospital started to set up its Facebook page, the organization found that one of its patients had already set up a page in its name to network with other teen patients.

## THE BENEFITS OUTWEIGH THE RISKS

Some fear that the simple act of setting up a weblog or other social networking site will invite a flood of unpleasant comments. However, the organizations described in the online book companion have found the opposite to be true. If you provide outlets that are easily accessible to everyone, any unpleasant comments will be mixed in with all the good things people have to say about the quality of care and service your organization provides. In addition, site moderators or the community can correct or remove inappropriate content, and all users have the option of commenting on what another user posts. And, perhaps more important, a negative post can expose problems of which the organization may not have been aware and can lead it to address these issues.

Social media, like all communication tools, have recognizable barriers and risks, but these can easily be overcome by forethought and planning. The greatest barrier for many healthcare organizations is their culture. Organizations and leaders who excel at innovation, transparency, collaboration, and communication will likely experience fewer challenges and less resistance. However, each organization's culture will need to be acknowledged, and leaders will want to invest sufficient time to work through concerns.

## PRIVACY AND SECURITY

An important concern in the adoption of a social media tool is that of protecting the privacy and security of information being shared. A thorough review of the intended use, audience, and tool must involve an evaluation of the tradeoff between privacy and the value of the information expected in return.

- Compliance policies should be reviewed and updated as needed to incorporate privacy and security protections related to new media. Just as policies have been put in place for keeping patient-identifiable information from being included in unsecured emails or left out in the open on counters or at fax machines, they are also needed to ensure that patient-identifiable information is not included in social networking posts.
- Organizations should update their policies defining and addressing the release of confidential, personal, proprietary, or otherwise sensitive information to include social media. In some cases, decisions may be made to balance the release of strategic information with the quality of the information expected in return.
- Whether traditional or new media, standards of care and professional judgment and responsibility still apply. Policies and guidelines for employees, contractors, independent practitioners, and others affiliated with your organization should address privacy, ground rules, and behavior standards.
- Participation in some forms of social networking may warrant user agreements.
- A specific decision to keep one's personal life and friends separate from one's professional persona and connections may also be appropriate.

Organizations should implement guidelines and policies on confidentiality and train employees, contractors, physicians, and others to understand and agree with expectations for use of the tools (AT&T 2008). These policies should include provisions for monitoring progress, ensuring moderation, and making adjustments as needed. This can include periodic reevaluations of how and when information is released as social media tools improve, confidence in security mechanisms flourishes, and trust among users grows.

A HIMSS Vantage Point survey (December 2009) revealed that 36 percent of organizations have policies outlining appropriate use of social technologies by employees. While 2 percent reported not having such policies, 17 percent reported plans to develop them in the future.

## TECHNOLOGICAL BARRIERS

Insufficient technology may be at least a temporary barrier for those with limited bandwidth or those in rural or isolated areas. This may be especially true of social networking tools that involve sharing large files, such as digital images. These organizations should determine whether they will have sufficient capacity for large video and picture files before investing time and energy developing an online video library or digital photo collection.

## LEGAL RISKS

According to Robert Coffield (2009), social media tools are so new that few legal decisions have been issued regarding their use—and there are no known laws. At this point, attorneys can only speculate as they analyze the law and social media, with the exception of discovery litigation, where there is significant activity. Attorneys are asking for—and accessing—more information from plaintiffs bringing claims against defendants. The content they find in social media portals can be valuable and can lead to other discoverable items.

Attorneys are also closely monitoring live "tweeting" of surgeries and other procedures, which is particularly interesting from the medical malpractice standpoint and raises the question of whether the information tweeted will be useful if future litigation arises.

*The sooner you are engaged and appropriately responding, the better.*

As with any new tool, a systematic, scientific-method approach, such as Plan-Do-Check-Act (PDCA), can reduce risks by focusing the organization on finding the right tool to meet the specific need of the appropriate audience. This type of disciplined approach will help the organization identify and quantify the value of each social media project. However, some healthcare organizations may find that the discussion has already turned from the need for a quantifiable return on investment to the use of social media being just another cost of doing business.

Healthcare leaders find that it is better to be proactive, address the barriers, and find creative ways to manage the challenges of these new communication tools. Those who ignore social media risk the unnecessary spread of potentially harmful and uncontested information and damage to their organizations' reputations and customer relations. The sooner you are engaged and appropriately responding, the better.

CHAPTER 4

# Weblogs

Weblogs, or blogs, are websites made up of entries—commonly known as posts—listed in chronological order. Posts can be categorized and viewed by topic or by date, and readers are free to comment on the original post or on the comments of other readers.

## WHY BLOG?

This form of social media provides an extraordinary opportunity for interactive online dialogue and the cataloging, journaling, and archiving of digital content. Blogs keep stakeholders updated and informed on construction and capital campaign projects, workplace issues, performance improvement initiatives, community health events, patient support groups, news, awards ▸

and recognition, policy changes, patient satisfaction, and personnel changes.

Blogs require a time investment, but they are one of the best places for a health professional or healthcare organization to start with social networking. According to Lisa Wehr, CEO of OneUpWeb, a blog gives healthcare leaders an opportunity to crack the door wider and make the transition to social media smoother by offering more control over the message. It serves as a tool to prove the concept and gain buy-in from others in the organization.

Most blogs include a blogroll (on the sidebar) that reflects the blogger's areas of interest. However, blogrolls also have other important functions.

- They provide readers with easy links to other sites that may be of interest and may help drive traffic to fellow bloggers.
- Fellow bloggers usually reciprocate by including your blog on their blogroll, and this broadens your audience by driving new readers to your site.
- Potential bloggers can use a blogroll to explore existing blogs in their area(s) of interest and stimulate ideas for their own.

Once you decide to create a weblog, you must decide

1. whether the blog will be sponsored by your organization or will be your personal/professional blog and
2. whether your blog will be public (accessible via the Internet) or private (accessible only via an intranet or otherwise secured).

If your blog represents your healthcare organization, decide on a tone and a style that supports the organization's brand, the blog's intended use, and the target audience. If you start instead with a personal or professional blog, be mindful of your organization's culture and discuss your approach with your supervisor, if appropriate.

## THE BLOG CONVERSATION

Comments are replies to your posts and the best indicator that you have successfully started a conversation. Weblog readers don't usually comment on every post they read, and some may never comment. Those who do leave comments likely have received something of value from the post and in turn want to contribute to the conversation or to build on the information. It is customary to allow comments, but be proactive: Establish a plan for responding to negative views and protect your reputation and brand by monitoring for violations of your site's standards.

In some cases, a comment left on your post will be spam that is only meant to promote another's site or product (similar to a grocer writing a letter to the editor that serves no purpose other than to promote his holiday sale). Most blogging services offer spam-blocking software; use this to monitor your posts and delete anything that looks like a sales pitch or doesn't fit with the content of your site.

If you are not interested in the online conversation, don't enable comments when you set up the site. Since those already familiar with the technology will expect to be able to leave comments, explain your decision in your first post or in a sidebar note. The three hospitals of MediSys Health Network, Inc., in New York use a weblog to publish the Medisys Pulse Newsletter (medisys.typepad.com). This weblog doesn't accept comments but still efficiently communicates news from each hospital to anyone who may have an interest—and this may be enough to meet the system's needs.

## BLOGGING SOLUTIONS

Weblogs can accommodate **widgets**, digital images, audio, the organization's logo, and links to other social media or websites to help enhance the attractiveness of the site. They can also accommodate advertising, but this should only be added after careful consideration of how your community and readers might perceive it.

---

**Web widget**—A portable chunk of code that can be installed and executed within any separate HTML-based Web page by an end user without requiring additional compilation. Other terms used to describe Web widgets include *gadget, badge, module, webjit, capsule, snippet, mini,* and *flake*. Widgets often take the form of on-screen tools (e.g., clocks, event countdowns, auction tickers, stock market tickers, or flight arrival or daily weather information).

---

Hospital CEOs are beginning to adopt blogging technology in greater numbers. Users include

- Marty Bonick, FACHE, president and CEO of Jewish Hospital and Frazier Rehab Institute in Louisville, Kentucky, who writes his personal blog, "Hospital Life" (www.hlifeblog.com), on life, work, and everything in between to enhance communications with his staff;
- Chuck Dorman, FACHE, CEO of Wilmington Veterans Affairs Medical Center, who uses his blog on the hospital's intranet to enhance his communications with staff; and
- Paul Levy, president and CEO of Beth Israel Deaconess Medical Center in Boston, who shares his thoughts about hospitals, medicine, and healthcare issues on his blog, "Running a Hospital" (http://runningahospital.blogspot.com).

Hospitals and other healthcare organizations can also host weblogs for patients undergoing unexpected or long-term treatment to help them keep family and friends informed and engaged. One study found that more than 10 percent of discussions on patient weblogs are dedicated to messages of appreciation, gratitude, and the positive effect of receiving emotional support (Langshur 2008).

Blogs are also helpful in brainstorming complicated health policy or strategies and gathering public input or feedback. In 2007, the U.S. Department of Health and Human Services (HHS) used a blog to convene an online leadership forum on pandemic preparedness, which brought together influential leaders from the business, faith, civic, and healthcare sectors to discuss how to convince Americans that they should prepare for a possible influenza pandemic and how to do it. The results were incorporated into operational plans to improve the public's response to current threats.

## GETTING STARTED

The most important question to ask before you start a blog is "who will keep it current and regularly add relevant content?" To keep the content fresh and interesting, this person or group will need to

- decide on topics for posts;
- write the posts in a conversational manner that engages readers;
- build trust and confidence;
- move readers to take action;

- monitor comments and **trackbacks**;
- add widgets, badges, links, and other applications to enhance the reader's experience; and
- if public, promote the weblog through other sites and search engines.

---

**Trackback**—One of three types of linkbacks, which are methods for Web authors to request notification when a user links to one of their documents. This enables authors to keep track of who is linking, and therefore referring, to their articles.

---

It is ideal to invest in your own domain, and some blogging services like Typepad (www.typepad.com/business/benefits.html) offer this option. A blogging service is especially attractive if you are interested in starting out with just a pilot or if you lack the expertise to design and build your own blog. When you use a blogging service provider and don't secure your own domain, you risk losing the links and content built over time if the provider shuts down or you want to change providers. However, services can teach you to navigate a blog and get started quickly with little, if any, out-of-pocket cost.

## MANAGING YOUR REPUTATION

Healthcare organizations work hard to maintain their reputations, so minimizing the risk of inappropriate content appearing on your blog (or other social networking site) is vital. There are two ways to ensure that blog content is appropriate for the organization's desired purpose (Thielst 2007):

1. Identify a moderator who can establish and apply the blog's use and posting policies. This person should regularly review the posted content and remove anything unsuitable, including personal attacks, foul language, and spam. The blog can also be set up to accept comments only from registered users or to post comments only after they have been reviewed and approved.
2. Include your policies and expectations for the blog on the site and establish a self-policing blog, where readers accept responsibility for reporting, removing, and/or correcting inappropriate content.

Mayo Clinic (2009a, 2009b) posts great examples of blog commenting guidelines for the general readership and for its employees on its site. Another option is to include a disclaimer, such as the one on the Children's Medical Center (2009) weblog "From the Red Balloon":

> This site is not written by a physician and is meant only to entertain and inspire compelling conversation. For more information about health-related topics discussed here, please consult with your child's physician.
>
> Children's Medical Center is not responsible for user-generated content or comments.

## TIPS FOR BLOGGERS

If your blog is visible and open for commenting by the public, consider the following suggestions:

- Tell your stories and invite readers to get to know your healthcare organization.
- Invite posts from those in your organization who can share unique expertise and knowledge.
- Announce awards, recognition, milestones reached, and other timely and relevant information.
- Follow the editorial calendar for your traditional media strategies, and include a link to your weblog posts, thus providing additional information in various formats.
- Educate readers on new developments, medical advances, best practices, and changing regulations or laws.
- Solicit feedback and survey readers, and then incorporate this information into your performance-improvement program.
- Set up a disclaimer or an explanation of your comments policy in the sidebar.
- Create a blogroll and include other blogs that might interest your readers.

Once your blog is established and you have started posting, promote it by doing the following:

- Include a link on your website, e-mail signature lines, brochures, and other collateral materials.
- Invite your employees, physicians, volunteers, and their family and friends to join the conversation.
- Submit your blog to blog directories, Technorati (technorati.com), healthcare aggregators like

TrustedMD (trusted.md), and search engines.

- Post relevant comments on other blogs or social networking sites with a link back to your blog.
- Allow (enable) trackbacks to your posts.
- Ask other bloggers to include your link in their blogrolls.
- Send out press releases to your local traditional media (radio, TV, newspapers, and newsletters) to promote your organization's entry into the blogosphere.

Blogs can also facilitate conversations among employees, physicians, volunteers, medical and other health professionals, students, and governance and other groups on secured networks. Depending on your purpose and the audience, apply the same suggestions provided for public blogs, as appropriate.

CHAPTER 5

# Microblogs

**Microblogs** are real-time tools for posting short comments from a computer or handheld device. In the case of Twitter (twitter.com), the most popular microblog today, comments are limited to 140 characters. These short person-to-person(s) communications, or "tweets," usually communicate news, announcements, event reminders, information about products and services, or simply what the user is doing at the moment.

---

**Microblogging**—A form of multimedia blogging that allows users to publish brief text updates or micromedia such as photos or audio clips, either to be viewed by anyone or to be viewed by a restricted group chosen by the user. These messages can be submitted by a variety of means, including text messaging, instant messaging, e-mail, digital audio, or the Web. ▶

---

A "re-tweet" is sending out a tweet from someone you follow to those who follow you. This capability circulates the most exceptional bursts of information, with an accompanying link to the details, providing an average person with the power to reach the masses with his or her message.

## THE GROWTH OF MICROBLOG USE

In May 2009, Nielsen reported that the time people spend on social networking and blog sites increased 82 percent from 2008 and that the average time per person increased 67 percent. Of the various media, Twitter was identified as the fastest-growing Web brand, increasing 1,448 percent, from 1.2 million unique visitors in May 2008 to 18.2 million in 2009. The average time per person on Twitter increased 175 percent, from 6 minutes and 19 seconds in May 2008 to 17 minutes and 21 seconds in May 2009, as illustrated in Exhibit 5.1. Although Twitter's trend could begin to level off, we can expect to see other applications for the technology and continued growth in microblogging.

As we have seen in the news, hospitals are providing real-time updates on surgeries and during disaster events. Twitter helped Innovis Health send out communications

**Exhibit 5.1: Twitter.com Time per Person Growth**

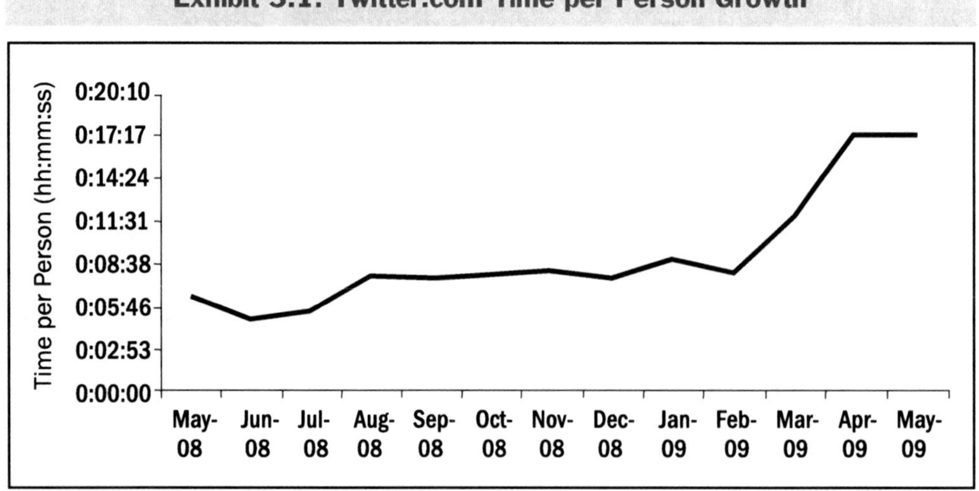


SOURCE: The Nielsen Company (2009).

and updates during a disaster after traditional mechanisms failed, and it increased awareness about living organ donation during a father–son kidney donation and transplant at Children's Medical Center in Dallas. But patients and their families may also be tweeting about the birth or death of a loved one and their experiences while in the hospital or waiting for an appointment. Healthcare leaders need to be aware of these tweets because they are showing up on search engine findings.

The popularity of microblogging could be explained by a study that finds a link between the speed of thought and a person's mood (Pronin and Wegner 2008). The researchers found an increase in positive mood when subjects thought quickly rather than slowly, and they postulate that the rapid growth of microblogging could be connected to the energy, motivation, and creativity users get from the short bursts of a microblog post.

According to iCrossing, the real value of microblogging is that the ordinary person can stay in contact with the extraordinary, and therefore the tool presents new



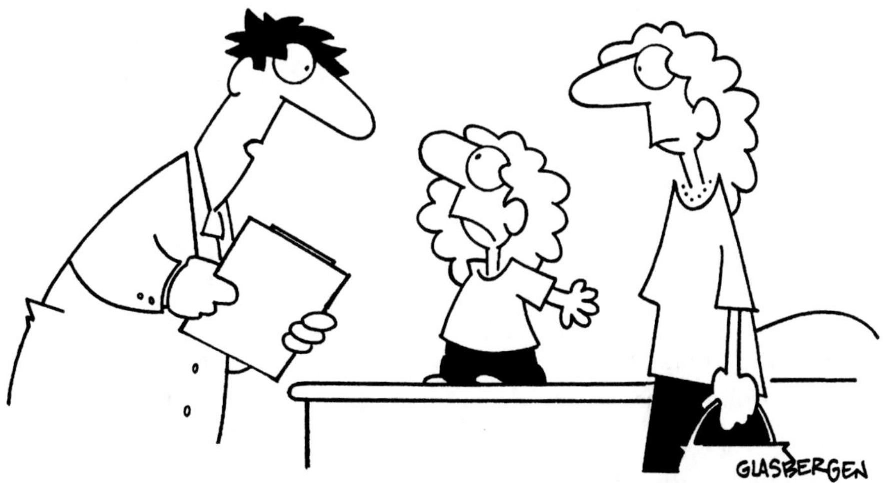


"Could you please stop Twittering your friends that I smell like salami. It's bad for my business!"

engagement opportunities (Harrington 2009). In business, microblogs are used to draw attention to a promotion or sponsorship, to listen and respond to consumer conversations, and to create new customer support channels to build affinity with the people who drive and embody the organization's brand.

## MICROBLOGS AND HEALTHCARE

The weblog VizEdu (2009) provides a great visual presentation of healthcare uses for microblogs. It reviews potential Twitter uses, such as

- physicians communicating with their patients;
- doctors helping those trying to keep track of them;
- hospitals monitoring what patients, doctors, staff, and others are saying about them; and
- medical devices tweeting blood pressure, blood sugar levels, or fetal heart beats.

The presentation highlights Kickbee (portfolio.menscher.com/itp/honeycomb), a device that uses Twitter as a platform to record and transmit "kick" messages to fathers as mobile phone text messages when the device is strapped onto a pregnant mother's belly and the little one gets active.

Phil Baumann, RN (2009), created a list of 140 healthcare uses for Twitter on his weblog, "Health Is Social," and my favorites are

- emitting and documenting critical lab and biomedical device values to nurses and physicians,
- bed and census management and monitoring,
- shift-bidding for nurses and other healthcare professionals,
- mood tracking and check-ins for patients with psychiatric disorders,
- prescription management (refill reminders, ordering, and notifications that prescriptions are ready for pickup),
- posting brief nursing assessments to a patient's electronic health record,
- reporting medical device malfunctions and alerting for routine preventive maintenance,
- reporting and documenting pain,
- tracking equipment/medication/supply recall notices, and
- disaster alerts and response communications.

For the day-to-day business of healthcare, microblog services like

Yammer (www.yammer.com) and Co-Tweet (cotweet.com) offer a simple way for employees and others to connect and share by posting short messages. These internal business communication tools provide a platform for corporate social networking and discussion.

Twitter and most other microblog accounts are free, and it is a good idea to sign on, if only to secure the name of your organization for your use. In addition to communicating out, healthcare organizations can use tracking tools that monitor microblog conversations and report posts that include a reference to your organization. Once you know what people are tweeting about your organization, you can respond, as appropriate.

## GETTING STARTED

Once your account is established, you can start following others who are posting by searching for people or organizations of interest or typing in the addresses of those you know. You can also join any of the groups of microbloggers that continually form around common interests.

You are likely to start being followed as soon as your account is established and you send out your first post, but monitor your followers, and use the blocking feature to prevent those who may present concerns. Accept friends and followers selectively on microblogs or any other social networking site. Following another user's tweets could be perceived as an endorsement or approval of their messages. Anne Arundel Medical Center has addressed this concern with a disclaimer on its Twitter profile (@AAMC) that "a follow is not an endorsement."

Promote your public microblog account address in your collateral materials, on your social media and websites, and in correspondence. If you establish a corporate microblog, promote it internally with those who will be involved. At a minimum, establish an account that allows you to easily communicate with your employees, physicians, vendors, and other key partners during an emergency. Include this communication tool in your emergency operations plan, and distribute the account address with other emergency information.

There are three options for following and sending tweets:

- Sign on to your account at the microblog site to send and follow tweets.

- Download a widget (application) to send and follow tweets from your computer's desktop.
- Download a widget (application) to send and follow tweets using your smartphone/PDA.

In addition to a short message, include links to websites, weblogs, or social networking sites with more detailed information, including text, photos, video, and podcasts. Many of the microblogging sites use TinyURL, which takes long website addresses and assigns them shorter URLs so that you have more characters left for the message to promote the link.

When you receive an exceptional post that is worth sharing, re-tweet it to those who follow you.

Periodically search for any posts that reference your organization, or use browsers like Tweetdeck (tweetdeck.com/beta) to customize your Twitter (and Facebook) experiences and manage tweets, track search results, and monitor what people are saying about you.

CHAPTER 6

# Social Networking Sites

Social networking services, such as MySpace, Facebook, LinkedIn, and others, allow users to network and share information with "friends" or "connections."

With 144.3 million unique visitors, Facebook (www.facebook.com) was the top global social networking destination in May 2009—for the seventh month in a row. May 2009 also marked the fifth month in a row that Facebook was the top social networking spot in the United States, with 75.4 million unique visitors—a 190 percent increase from a year earlier (Nielsen 2009b). And the fastest growing user segment consists of those aged 35 or older. (See Exhibit 6.1.)

Facebook and other social networking sites allow the user to create a digital identity and to communicate with others who share the same interests. As we have seen happen in microblogging, Facebook users are forming and joining groups around common interests, issues, professions, diseases, and conditions to broaden their networks. ▶

**Exhibit 6.1: Facebook's Growth in Global* Audience Numbers**

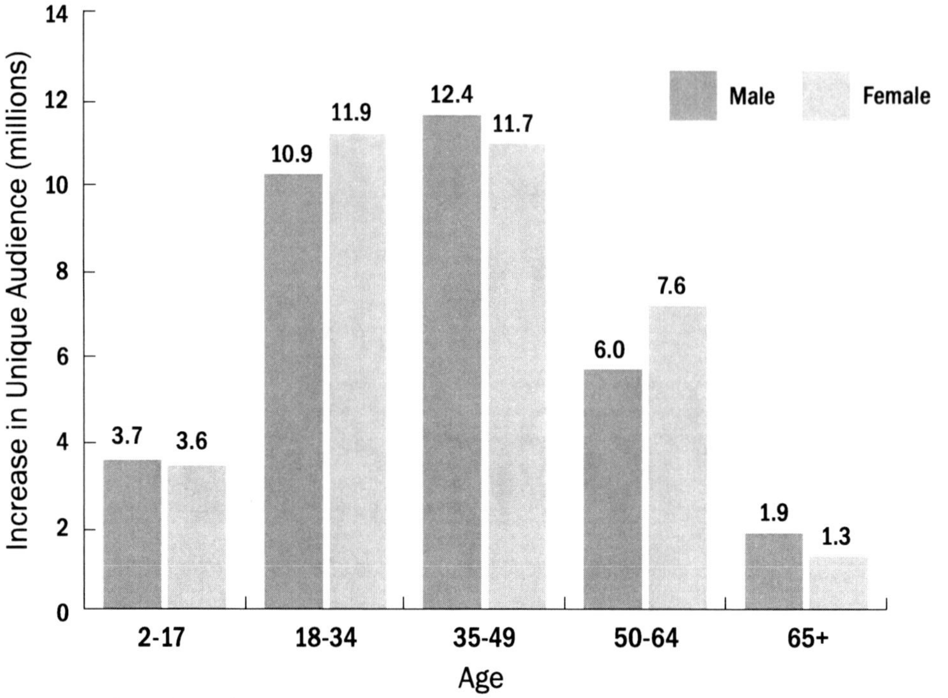

SOURCE: Nielsen (2009a).
NOTE: Between December 2007 and December 2008 there was a 3.7 million global increase in the number of 2- to 17-year-old males visiting Facebook. *Global* refers to Australia, Brazil, Switzerland, Germany, Spain, France, Italy, the United Kingdom, and the United States only.

Another social networking site, popular with professionals and business leaders, is LinkedIn (www.linkedin.com). This site is also seeing huge growth, 137 percent over 2008 (Nielsen 2009a). LinkedIn users can build online networks through "connections," or people they know, and join professionally oriented groups sponsored by alumni associations, professional organizations, and businesses of which they may be members or customers. Other LinkedIn groups bring together individuals with common interests, such as

- pharmaceutical and medical professionals,
- healthcare supply chain professionals,
- healthcare management engineers, and
- healthcare physician practice managers.

On any social networking site, you should allow only people you know and trust—people with whom you feel comfortable sharing information and contacts—to join your network. Wisely select connections and friends and, if necessary, maintain separate accounts for your personal and professional personae.

Respect and incorporate traditional boundaries when applying these communication and collaboration tools. Consider doctor–patient relationship concerns and employee–supervisor boundaries. Your reputation depends on it, so closely monitor your message and ensure that it fits with your audience.

A recent article about these conflicts includes a cautionary e-mail from a dean of medical education to students and faculty on the subject of social networking (Jain 2009):

> Caution is recommended . . . in using social networking sites such as Facebook or MySpace. Items that represent unprofessional behavior that are posted by you on such networking sites reflect poorly on you and the medical profession. Such items may become public and could subject you to unintended exposure and consequences.

## THE EFFECTS OF SOCIAL NETWORKING ON PHYSICIANS AND THEIR PATIENTS

In healthcare environments, social networking is most significantly affecting the medical community. Of physicians in the United States, 88 percent report that the Internet is essential to their practice, and 60 percent, largely younger female primary care physicians, are interested in using online physician communities, like Sermo (www.sermo.com) and Physician Connect (www.medscape.com/connect) to share information, ideas, opinions, and experiences with fellow physicians (Manhattan Research 2009).

Social networking sites blend comments made by traditional opinion leaders with comments from other physicians, who can agree, disagree, or even challenge the opinion leaders in real time.

A recent study reports that approximately 53 percent of nursing schools and 45 percent of medical schools are using social networking tools to enhance instruction (Lemley and Burnham 2008). The tools most commonly used are blogs, wikis, videocasts, and podcasts. As Exhibit 6.2 shows, practicing physicians and

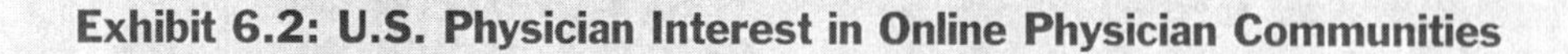
Exhibit 6.2: U.S. Physician Interest in Online Physician Communities

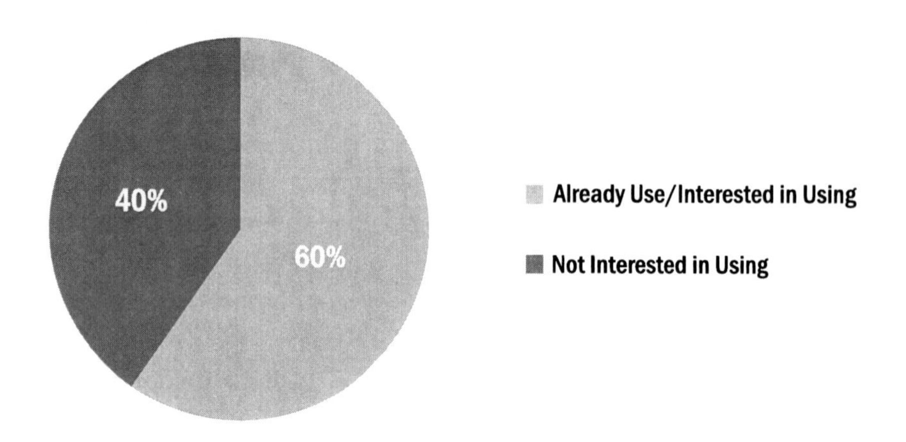


SOURCE: Adapted from Manhattan Research (2009).

other healthcare leaders are also using these new tools in virtual interactive conferences or meetings.

Almost a quarter of online health searchers turn to online content created by others in similar situations or to online social communities where they can share experiences about a disease or condition (Langshur 2008). Popular health-oriented social networking sites include the following:

- PatientsLikeMe (www.patientslikeme.com)—individuals who share a diagnosis.
- GroupLoop (www.grouploop.org) —teens (and their families) dealing with a cancer diagnosis.
- ChangeHealthcare (www.changehealthcare.com)—individuals, employees, and employers who share, track, and compare their experiences with providers, other health services, insurance, health issues, bills and cost, etc.
- One Recovery's (www.onerecovery.com) platform helps people recover from addiction. In 2010, Aetna became the first insurer to provide its members with an online support network and mobile tools to help them remain sober.

Some physicians are using Hello Health (www.hellohealth.com), a Facebook-like platform that incorporates technology—from instant messaging to video chat—to enhance the doctor–patient relationship. It helps physicians blend online communication with traditional home or office visits to give patients personal attention when and how they want it. The option of a virtual practice is attractive to many physicians and patients and also to employers looking to offer their employees convenient healthcare, provide company doctors on demand, and minimize the number of days off from work.

## THE EFFECTS OF SOCIAL NETWORKING ON THE WORKPLACE

Employers struggling to recruit healthcare professionals are going online where people gather—LinkedIn, Facebook, and other social networking sites. A healthcare organization's Facebook profile and page can

- convey why your facility is a great place to work,
- help identify candidates and promote opportunities,
- link readers to the job opportunities on your website, and
- include testimonials from current or former employees.

Forty-five percent of employers use social networking sites for pre-employment screening (CareerBuilder 2009). Of 2,600 hiring managers who responded to a survey, 35 percent found content that caused them to not hire a candidate, and 18 percent found content that caused them to make an offer to a candidate. Some of the methods hiring managers use to find information about a candidate that may not be included in his or her resume include

- viewing their Facebook pages and friends (26%),
- viewing their LinkedIn profile and connections (26%),
- viewing their MySpace pages (21%),
- searching blogs and their posts (11%), and
- following their tweets (7%).

Social networking tools can also be used to create workspaces on an organization's secured intranet site that can facilitate employee or medical staff activities or present issues for discussion or debate. Residents and other students can use these sites to interact and share their individual experiences, and project teams and employees can use them to share ideas and best practices and provide support.

The most effective ways to engage employees in improving their health and well-being is to connect those with similar interests and promote available resources. Employers are using online social networking tools that are already widely available for this purpose. One example is BeWell@Stanford (Wellsphere 2009), which was designed to improve the health and well-being of the Stanford University community (30,000 students, faculty, staff, and area residents). This site provides members with personalized information, wellness resources and activities, and a forum to meet like-minded people and form groups for support, advice, and encouragement.

## SOCIAL NETWORKING IN 3D

A different form of social networking site uses simulated environments where users can interact using avatars (user-created, 3D, digital representations). A survey of the popular site Second Life identified 68 healthcare-related services sponsored by real-world hospitals, healthcare consumer groups, and government organizations (Beard et al. 2009). The authors found that healthcare organizations use these platforms for education, research, and disease surveillance. Patients can use the sites to gain insight into medical procedures and processes—for example by virtually experiencing a mammogram or navigating a hospital's virtual ward.

The survey also found that the principal aim of the activities was patient education or increased awareness about health issues, but other goals included providing support, training, and marketing uses. A few sites were built to conduct research in the virtual world or to recruit participants for real-life research. The authors concluded that behaviors from virtual worlds can translate to the real world and affect users' real-life behaviors.

The Centers for Disease Control (CDC) has used Whyville, a popular site with tweens (ages 10 to 13), to educate kids on hand washing, seasonal flu, and vaccinations. The CDC launched Why-Pox lab (http://i.whyville.net/smmk/virus/whypoxLab) to teach kids about the spread of infectious diseases and then followed up with WhyFlu campaigns. During the 2007–2008 WhyFlu campaign, they encouraged kid avatars to get their flu shots and virtually vaccinated more than 41,000 people before unleashing a virus that sent many avatars off to a clinic for treatment. The virtual flu virus spread though the Whyville world to those who had not gotten the vaccination. Infection was represented by virtual sneezes and spots showing up on avatars' faces, interrupting the kids' online conversations.

Social networks and virtual world technologies are also being used to create orientation, education, and training programs for patients, physicians, and other healthcare professionals. Healthcare organizations can reach new audiences and can improve their effectiveness by using the interaction of multiple participants in different roles to test responses to actions or allowing them to see their avatars perform the participants' chosen behaviors. Examples of healthcare organizations' use of these 3D tools include the following:

- Cleveland Clinic Lerner College of Medicine (www.clevelandclinic.org/cclcm) partnered with Second Life to create mock situations where psychology students can conduct medical history interviews with virtual patients controlled by professors (Cleveland.com 2009).
- Stanford University's Center for Immersive and Simulation-Based Learning (2009) has created virtual worlds in its School of Medicine, such as the virtual emergency department, which is used to train residents and students using different trauma scenarios. (See Exhibit 6.3.)
- HotZone uses a virtual world to train teams of first responders to a chemical and explosive attack on triage, evacuation, decontamination, and identifying the source of the chemical release (Noblis 2007).
- Children's Memorial Hospital created a virtual replica of its hospital to conduct realistic disaster training exercises without risks to patients.

## GETTING STARTED

Healthcare organizations should have discussions with employees and others in the workplace about acceptable behavior on social networking sites, especially if their actions could reflect on the reputation of the organization.

If your organization creates a social networking site, clearly explain the terms and conditions of use and encourage community policing for inappropriate content. Behavior in any social network should be respectful and appropriate, and the expectations of the owners of the site and the community should be clearly defined.

Some healthcare organizations start with one or two Facebook pages for individual departments or service lines before building others and reserve the main Facebook page for community relations and media content. Organizations that take this route should establish a clear plan and goals for each page.

Any social networking requires staff time for setting up, adding content, linking, and monitoring. Out-of-pocket costs, if any, are minimal for most public sites, but costs for establishing social networks on your intranet or creating computer-based simulated environments (virtual worlds) can be significant. However, depending on the purpose of the project and expected return, these costs may be acceptable.

**Exhibit 6.3: A Screenshot from Stanford University School of Medicine's Virtual World**

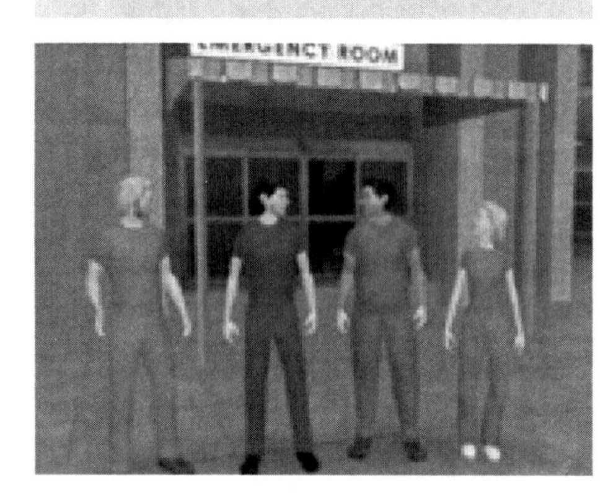

SOURCE: Stanford University School of Medicine, Center for Immersive and Simulation-based Learning. 2009. Reprinted with permission.

CHAPTER 7

# Podcasts

A podcast is a digital audio file distributed via websites, weblogs, or social networking sites. Podcasts can be downloaded to a smart phone, an MP3 player, an iPod, or the listener's computer. They are a progressive way to present your health organization's brand, educate people, and reach broader audiences. They are excellent for communicating with those who prefer an auditory format (OneUpWeb 2006), including

- the visually impaired,
- frequent travelers,
- those whose schedules or work habits limit the time they spend online,
- those with limited reading skills, ▸

- commuters, and
- multitaskers.

As Exhibit 7.1 illustrates, the podcast audience is expected to reach 17 percent of all Internet users by 2013. Some of these listeners will be those e-patients currently going online to find information on hospitals, doctors, and insurance/payers.

Healthcare organizations create podcasts to build relationships and strengthen their brands with the public, patients, employees, physicians, and other stakeholder groups. Listeners invite the message into their lives by downloading the audio file from the organization's intranet, website, or weblog, or another social networking site. Podcasts can also be pushed out to those who subscribe via **RSS** feeds to receive new releases. The result is on-demand, portable information with excellent tracking capabilities.

---

**RSS** (most commonly translated as "Really Simple Syndication")—A family of Web feed formats used to publish frequently updated works—such as blog entries, news headlines, audio, and video—in a standardized format. An RSS document (which is called a "feed," "Web feed," or

**Exhibit 7.1: U.S. Podcast Audience, 2008–2013, in Millions and Percent of Internet Users**

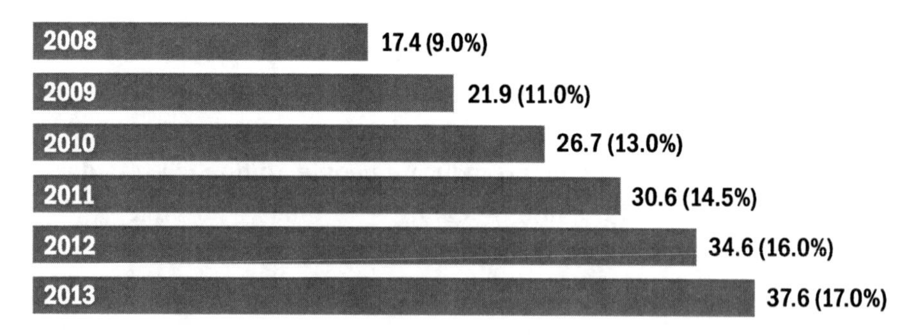


**Note: Internet users who download or stream at least one podcast per month**
**Note: 2009 through 2013 are projections.**

SOURCE: eMarketer (2009). Reprinted with permission.

"channel") includes full or summarized text, plus metadata such as publishing dates and authorship.

---

More physicians than average consumers are adopting this medium and a physician is more likely than the average 18- to 34-year-old male to own an iPod. This may be attributable to the fact that many physicians are constantly on the move. They have challenging work schedules, time limitations, and, in some cases, long commutes and frequent travel obligations.

## PODCAST USES

Podcasts can be used to distribute recorded interviews of your experts in the field (physicians, nurses, pharmacists, managers, executives, and other health professionals), content from presentations, and other audio recordings. Examples of uses, by audience category, include the following:

- Public
  - information about health conditions and diseases
  - prevention and safety tips
  - descriptions and facts about program and service offerings
  - press releases
  - newsletters
  - events calendars
  - comments on current issues
  - public service announcements/ advisories
  - annual reports
- Staff
  - employee orientation and updates
  - briefs on changing legislation, rules and regulations, and accreditation standards
  - review or overview of policies, procedures, plans, protocols, or guidelines
  - CEU or CME programs
  - employee or medical staff newsletters
  - employee handbook
  - clinical guidelines/protocols
- Patients
  - admit, pre-op/post-op, medication, and discharge instructions (to enhance what is provided in writing or exchanged in person)
  - review of billing policies and procedures or discount programs
  - welcome messages or introductions to nursing units or programs
  - description of patient rights
  - description of the compliance program

- Governing body:
  - board member orientation
  - briefs on changing legislation, rules and regulations, and accreditation standards
  - reviews of issues or proposed policies and plans on the next agenda
  - stories from patients, families, employees, physicians, volunteers, and others that demonstrate the effects of their service to the organization

## GETTING STARTED

For successful podcasts, you need people who can produce quality audio and attend to your organization's brand and image. Public distributions require more attention to protecting your reputation and image than do internal distributions. Podcast producers must be skilled with writing scripts or talking points, production, speaking, and directing audio content. The best practices for podcasts include the following:

- Speak clearly, in a pleasant voice, and at an appropriate tempo.
- Target the content to your audience.
- Ensure that the content fits with your brand.
- Preapprove the script or talking points.
- Make your podcasts easy to find and download.

Exhibit 7.2 illustrates the process that leads to a successful podcast. Whether you do it yourself or bring in a production company, you can improve the final product and save on costs by completing the following steps before recording (OneUpWeb 2006):

- Identify your target audience.
- Survey other podcasts.
- Develop a creative approach.
- Get management buy-in.
- Determine how you will promote your podcast.
- Source your production.
- Commit to regular production.
- Pencil in topics for identified podcasts.
- Develop a topical outline.
- Script as much as your format permits.

In addition to the main content of your podcasts, consider

- adding music or voice at the beginning and end (introduction/exit),

## Exhibit 7.2: OneUpWeb Podcast Cycle

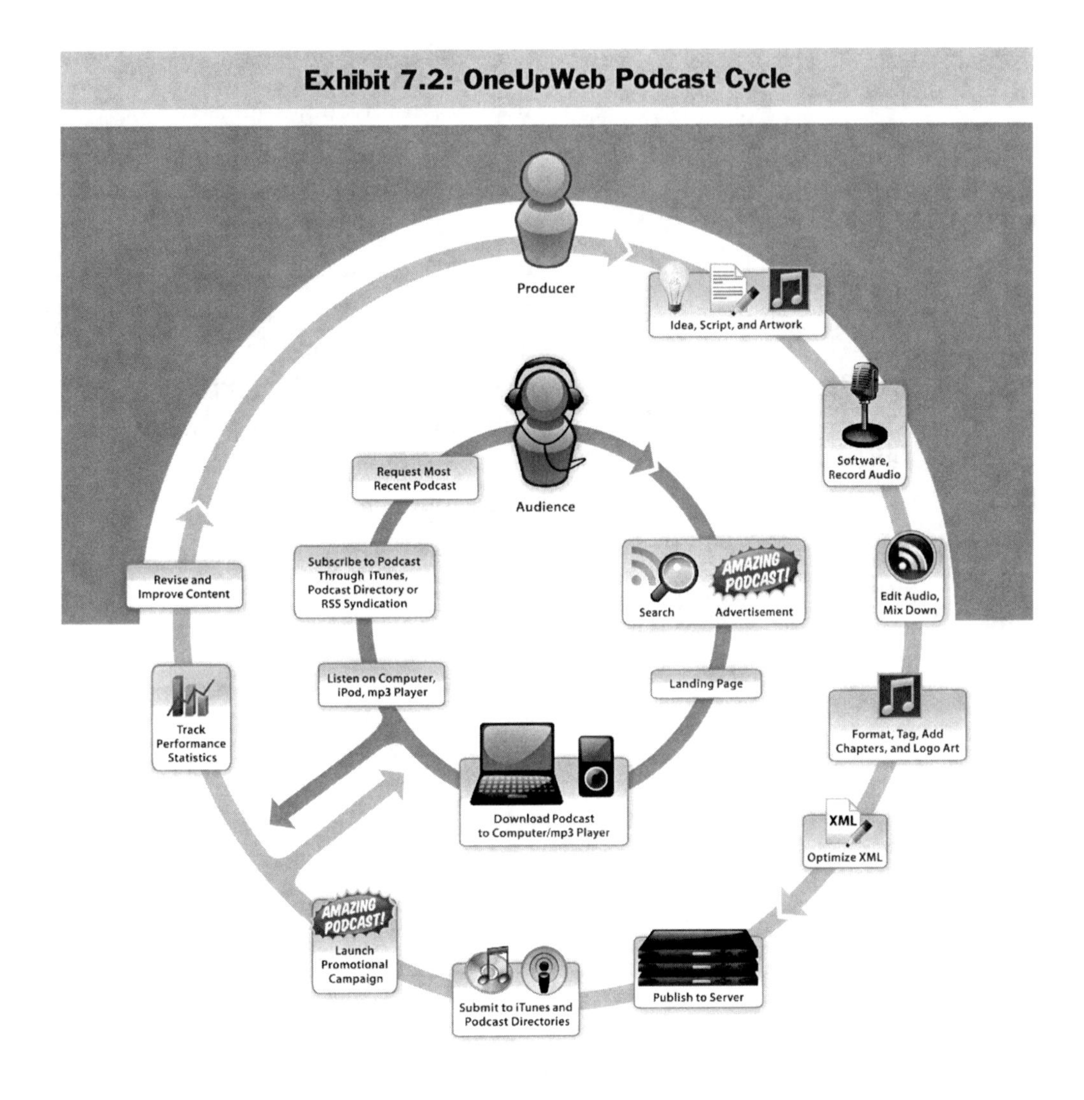


SOURCE: OneUpWeb (2006). Reprinted with permission.

- creating an XML feed to push the file out to directories,
- performing sound editing and evening, and
- installing software to track the number of downloads, sources of traffic, loyalty, and so on.

If you don't have the expertise to create your own content, consider prepared audio content available from organizations like Healthwise (www.healthwise.org/p_audio_library.aspx). Their user-friendly information on health, wellness, disease, and testing topics can be accessed through your website, weblog, or social networking site. Each topic begins with a general description of the condition and then reviews causes, symptoms, diagnosis, and treatment. You can easily brand the content by adding introductory and concluding messages from your organization and referring listeners to your intake or physician referral services.

CHAPTER 8

# The Wiki

A **wiki** is a website that uses content management software to allow users to read, edit, and search content posted by others or to add new content. The original and the modified content are stored as a comprehensive collection of knowledge. The collaboration and peer production capabilities offered by this social media tool usher us toward a "world where value creation will be fast, fluid, and persistently disruptive. A world where only the connected will survive" and "human skill, ingenuity, and intelligence [will be harnessed] more efficiently and effectively than anything we have witnessed previously" (Tapscott and Williams 2008).

---

**Wiki**—A website that uses wiki software, allowing users to create and edit any number of interlinked Web pages, using a simplified markup language or a ▶

WYSIWYG (what you see is what you get) text editor within the browser. Wikis are often used to create collaborative websites and to power community websites.

## WIKIPEDIA

Wikipedia (en.wikipedia.org/wiki/Main_Page), the best-known wiki, was created in 2001 as a reference website. Active contributors and visitors around the world continuously update the site's content. Wikipedia can be updated as soon as something happens that renders an entry out of date, rather than the months or years it takes to update printed encyclopedias or reference books. Substandard or disputed information is subject to removal, and mistakes can be corrected easily. Wikipedia has become one of the largest reference websites and attracts approximately 65 million visitors each month (Wikipedia 2009c).

Wikipedia provides opportunities for healthcare organizations and individuals with subject matter expertise to drive traffic to their websites, weblogs, and other online pages (Facebook, LinkedIn, etc.). Some healthcare organizations represented by Wikipedia articles include the following:

- Santa Paula Hospital (en.wikipedia.org/wiki/Santa_Paula_Hospital)
- Mayo Clinic (en.wikipedia.org/wiki/Mayo_clinic)
- Beth Israel Deaconess Medical Center (en.wikipedia.org/wiki/Beth_Israel_Deaconess_Medical_Center)
- Henry Ford Health System (en.wikipedia.org/wiki/Henry_Ford_Health_System)
- MD Anderson Cancer Center (en.wikipedia.org/wiki/MD_Anderson)

## WIKIS AND HEALTHCARE

Other wikis, such as AskDrWiki (http://askdrwiki.com/mediawiki/index.php?title=Main_Page) and MedPedia (www.medpedia.com), focus entirely on health and medical topics. These health information repositories are managed by contributing professionals and are gaining popularity with Internet users seeking information on health, medicine, and the body.

Wikis allow healthcare organizations to efficiently capture knowledge that already exists within the system. Workgroups and other collaborative teams dispersed among worksites or with alternate work schedules will find the technology especially attractive, because it can reduce the time needed for meetings or the number of e-mails circulating among the team. Team members can add, contribute to, and edit documents on the wiki.

The workforce of the future will be comfortable with the less costly and more effective peer-production and documentation methods wikis offer. Santa Clara Valley Health and Hospital System, a safety-net provider, is already realizing the benefits of collaboration and peer-production that result from using a wiki. Not surprisingly, adoption of the software in its residency program took off as soon as it was installed.

The effectiveness and success of a wiki project, as with any workplace initiative, depends on common principles, such as trust, clear goals, structure, discipline, and leadership.

## GETTING STARTED

Consider starting a Wikipedia article that describes your organization's history and contributions to the fields of healthcare and medicine. You may be surprised to find that your organization is already represented and that the page includes links to newspaper stories, research, and your website. However, the way this information is presented may not fit with the image you want to project. Review and monitor the content and contribute or edit, as needed, to ensure that it is accurate and fits with your strategy and branding.

Consider pilot projects using wiki software to test incentives, controls, quality, and trust before adopting it for broader use. Wikis to brainstorm, handle urgent projects, or create strategy, plans, and policies are ideal starting points to generate early wins and gain credibility and organizational buy-in.

Use wiki software in your workplace to stimulate creative thinking, engage employees and physicians, and capture the knowledge of your entire workforce and medical community. Consider a wiki to

- build a reference site of policies, procedures, plans, handbooks, protocols, guidelines, best practices, reports, regulations/legislation, and standards for employees, the medical staff, or patient groups;
- organize plans, policies, and other documentation for upcoming Joint Commission, state licensing, CLIA, CMS, Patient Rights, and other surveys or visits;

- organize troubleshooting or self-help manuals for IT (hardware and software), communications (two-way radio transceivers and cell, satellite, VOIP phones), biomedical equipment, patient home monitoring equipment, etc.;
- organize reference and training materials for staff education, new employee orientation, annual updates, compliance, safety, emergency preparedness, and competency testing;
- organize medical staff bylaws, rules, and regulations, clinical practice guidelines and protocols, member identification and credentialing for easy searching, and location of needed information;
- minimize the amount of face-to-face meeting time by having members discuss, comment on, and edit documents to be reviewed at the next meeting;
- track projects and document the extent of collaboration and multidisciplinary involvement; and
- organize patient education and training information and resources and provide patients with the opportunity to collaborate and share their knowledge and resources.

CHAPTER 9

# Social News and Bookmarking Sites

More and more, people get their news from the Internet. Online news sources include blogs, **social news sites**, and Web versions of traditional news media.

---

**Social news sites**—Websites that allow users to submit and vote on news stories or other links, thus determining which links are presented. The social news phenomenon has spawned a number of news aggregator sites, which collect and group articles based on Web interest, presenting users with a reflexive news feed. ▶

---

## SOCIAL NEWS

Social news sites allow users to submit news and press releases. Often, readers can vote on the value of the submitted content. The number of votes determines a news item's ranking, and those with the most votes get included on the front page of the site. Traditional media sources sometimes pick up on these stories for their broadcasts or publications.

General news sites, such as Digg (digg.com), promote conversation and filter information through the lens of the community. Like print newspapers, they have a front page (the homepage) and sections (categories), and they report information from many online sources, ranging from the most popular to the most obscure. Consumers of healthcare services receive news from these sites and use them to follow healthcare trends.

With 40 million unique visitors per month on Digg alone (see Exhibit 9.1), a story that readers find newsworthy could receive enough votes to move it to the front page for millions of others to see. The difference from traditional news media is that readers, not editors, collectively determine the value of the content.

Social news sites focused on health are just beginning to grow,

**Exhibit 9.1: Social News Sites: Unique Visitors by Month**

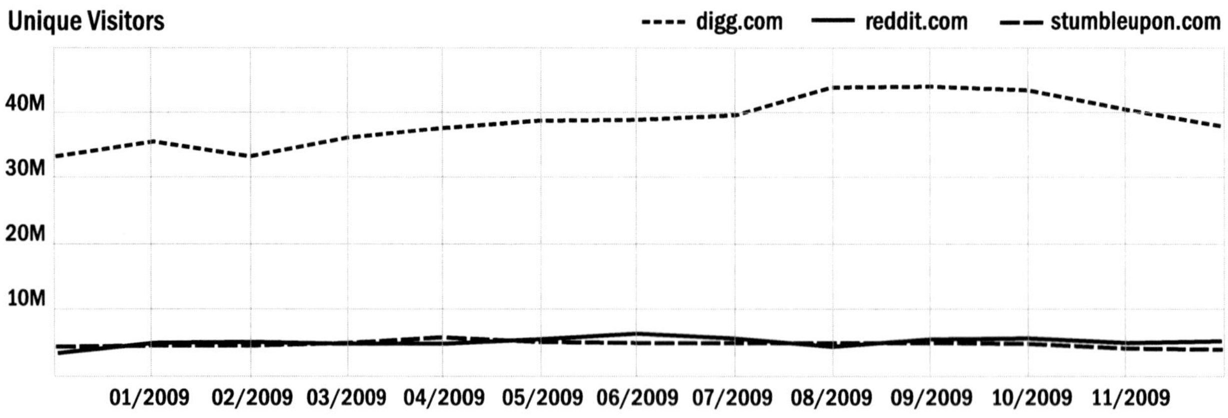

Unique Visitors
---- digg.com — reddit.com –– stumbleupon.com
40M
30M
20M
10M
01/2009 02/2009 03/2009 04/2009 05/2009 06/2009 07/2009 08/2009 09/2009 10/2009 11/2009

SOURCE: Compete (2009). Reprinted with permission.

as traditional industry media and healthcare organizations become aware of this opportunity to reach a broader audience. One healthcentric social news and voting site is Health Ranker (www.healthranker.com), with almost a million unique visitors in 2009. The site is dedicated to bringing the latest health news and health-related information to its readers. As healthcare social news sites mature, more news will be submitted by providers, plans, researchers, policymakers, and the public, and readers will cast their votes for the information they find most valuable.

## SOCIAL BOOKMARKING

**Social bookmarking** is a method for saving, organizing, searching, and sharing online links to pages on the Internet. It is often used in conjunction with social news and networking sites. The most popular general bookmarking site currently is Delicious (delicious.com). Health-oriented bookmarking sites include Health Pieces (www.healthbookmarks.com) and Healtheva (www.healtheva.com).

---

**Social bookmarking**—A method for Internet users to store, organize, search, and manage bookmarks of Web pages with the help of metadata, typically in the form of tags.

---

Bookmarks can be public, or they can be privately shared with specified people, groups, or networks (e.g., an intranet). Users can view bookmarks chronologically or by category or tags, or they can search them using a search engine. Some bookmarking services also report the number of users who have bookmarked an item, Web feeds for their lists of bookmarks, and other features, such as ratings or comments on bookmarks.

Social bookmarking provides a way to store, manage, and share links to important information. It can thus decrease the number of reference items circulated via e-mail.

## GETTING STARTED

- Consider using free press release distribution websites like Press Release Point (www.pressreleasepoint.com) to generate media visibility and maximize your organization's online presence. Prepare press releases on research findings, medical advances, awards and recognition, or timely health tips and information. This digital news can then be easily submitted to and picked up by social news sites. It can also be picked up by search engines to drive even more traffic to your website(s).

- Identify local or regional social news sites such as Noozhawk (www.noozhawk.com) and submit news on community events, changes to service offerings, or updates on construction or capital campaign projects.
- Bookmark
  - safety/disaster preparedness guides, checklists, resources, and training;
  - compliance guides and resources;
  - staff education resources and programs;
  - best practices;
  - news about your organization or staff; and
  - medical library and research references.

CHAPTER 10

# Photo and Video Sharing

The old saying that a picture is worth a thousand words highlights the potential benefit of combining visual media with text. Pictures help some people absorb data and can have a greater effect than text. And in some cases, the picture *says it all.*

Messages from healthcare environments can be complex—for example, when they relate to clinical conditions, disease processes, or courses of treatment. Videos and photos can clarify the information for laypeople (patients, their family members, or the public) or those with hearing or reading challenges. If the message is an appeal or a call to action, such as a blood drive announcement or a request for parents to bring children in for a vaccination, visible emotion or body language can strengthen its effect.

Photos and videos can be powerful tools when introducing a new charismatic CEO or physician to the community. The individual's appearance, body language, demeanor, mannerisms, and style as conveyed by these media can determine the first, and often the lasting, impression that will influence the relationships that follow.

**Photo sharing** began in the late 1990s with online photo finishing services and has evolved into permanent and centralized access to user photos and videos. Photo and video sharing tools allow users to upload and post digital photographs or videos on websites or weblogs and share them with other users, publicly or privately. Sites such as Flickr (www.flickr.com) provide users with various viewing options, including thumbnails, slideshows, and albums, and some offer desktop photo management capabilities.

---

**Photo sharing**—Publishing or transferring of a user's digital photos online, enabling the user to share them with others (publicly or privately). Websites and applications that allow the upload and display of images support this function.

---

Photoblogs and **video blogs** (vblogs), on the other hand, typically only display images chronologically. This form of blogging is popular among those in visual arts or anyone whose audience prefers a visual message. Sometimes visuals add additional information, and other times it is simply more attractive to readers. The combination of text, visual graphics, and audio data expands your ability to attract new audiences.

---

**Video blog**—(Sometimes shortened to vlog or vblog) A blog for which the medium is video. Entries are regular and often combine embedded video or a video link with supporting text, images, and other metadata. Video logs (vlogs) often take advantage of Web syndication to distribute video over the Internet, using the RSS or Atom syndication formats, for automatic aggregation and playback on mobile devices and personal computers.

---

## Sharing Photos and Videos in Healthcare

Popular video sharing sites such as YouTube (youtube.com) allow anyone to broadcast videos of themselves or others. Make sure you know what photos and videos are being posted online and tagged with the name of your organization.

Healthcare organizations that want to impart information to physicians should consider photo sharing or video sharing technology, since 83 percent of physicians report watching video. (Manhattan Research 2009). Photo and video sharing can be particularly useful for documenting rare and unusual medical conditions for teaching or reference purposes. It can also be used to educate and inform consumers, as WebMD does on its site with Bad Bugs and Their Bites (www.webmd.com/allergies/slideshow-bad-bugs) and Melanoma and Other Reasons to Shun the Sun (www.webmd.com/melanoma-skin-cancer/slideshow-sun-damaged-skin).

Historians managing the photographic history of a healthcare organization may find photo or video blogging useful. It can also be used to create a pool of photographs or video for staff to use in collateral materials, slide presentations, handouts, educational materials, and social media sites.

Intermountain Healthcare created an educational program using humorous videos on the topic of healthy habits to capture the attention of young audiences. Their LiVe program (intermountainlive.org/Pages/home.aspx) was created in response to a concern about childhood obesity. The health videos engage kids by using a medium that is familiar and attractive. The program is so successful that the video is now available through syndication (at healthmedia syndicate.com) for others to use in their markets. Syndication can help the producing organization recover a portion of its costs and allows other organizations to offer high-quality video to their communities at a much lower cost.

New, inexpensive digital cameras and video equipment are available and are ideal for most internal uses. They are easy to use and allow you to upload images to your website, weblog, social networking page, or YouTube page.

Investing in a more expensive, higher-quality video camera or reaching out to local production companies may be appropriate for formal or public projects. Just as with audio, video production companies can create XML feeds to push out to directories, dress up your final product (e.g., with music, a voice intro, or graphics), edit and even the sound, and add custom players or tracking systems so that you can monitor downloading activities, traffic, and subscriber loyalty.

## GETTING STARTED

Once you have started working with social media, think about how and where you can incorporate photographs, videos, and other visual media to enhance your posts and generate interest. If you already have a collection of videos or photographs, review it for possible additions to a video or photo library or blog.

As with podcasts for public distribution, determine whether any editing or dressing up is needed. Explore your options with local production companies or individuals who specialize in this type of production.

Use a video/photo cast to accomplish the following:

- Promote the practice of a new clinician or those with specialized knowledge and skills.
- Recognize employees of the month or distribute images of staff in action.
- Share messages from the CEO with those who don't have an opportunity to see him or her personally. The visual of a leader delivering news may be more powerful than the written word alone.
- Illustrate directions to the hospital or campus.
- Enhance instructions for use of a new piece of equipment or supply item.
- Illustrate signs and symptoms of diseases and conditions.
- Share day-to-day and special stories in and around the healthcare organization.
- Demonstrate new tools or techniques for staff, patient, and caregiver education and training.

CHAPTER 11

# Widgets and Other Tools

Widgets are mini applications that enhance an organization's website, weblog, or social networking site. They display an information arrangement, such as a window or a text box, that the user can change, providing a single interaction point for the direct manipulation of a given kind of data (Wikipedia 2009a).

## Business Applications

Some widgets, such as Slideshare (www.slideshare.net/widgets), allow users to upload, view, and share presentation files that can be added to websites, weblogs, and other social networking sites. Other widgets display your most recent Twitter or blog posts on your website, weblog, LinkedIn profile, or ▶

desktop. Some, like ChipIn (www.chipin.com/overview) can be used to collect money for a cause (staff parties, retirement gifts, nonprofit donations). Similar money-collection widgets such as PayPal Storefront (storefront.paypallabs.com) might be attractive to an auxiliary or hospital gift shop wanting to expand its customer base.

### Public Alerts and Information

The Centers for Disease Control (CDC) offers a variety of widgets (www.cdc.gov/Widgets) to help organizations, professionals, and individuals support its public outreach and educational goals. CDC's widgets include a swine flu graphic (in English and Spanish) with links to information and resources, the Flu IQ Interactive Quiz, and emergency text messages and alerts.

### Buttons and Badges

Other widgets include badges and buttons, which are graphical links to other sites. In healthcare, they are used to draw attention to an organization's site or raise awareness of issues. The code associated with the image can easily be added to websites, weblogs, and social networking sites, providing an attractive and easy link to additional information.

## WIDGETS FOR MOBILE DEVICES

Widgets can also bring online content to mobile devices. These widgets, or apps, allow users to read books and reference materials; receive news; manage their medications; log their vital signs, diet, and workouts; and perform other business and personal tasks.

Sites like Microsoft's Health Vault (www.healthvault.com) and Google Health (www.google.com/intl/en-US/health/about) allow users with a computer or mobile device to upload health information and data from hospitals, pharmacies, medical devices, and other sources to present a virtual personal health record. These free sites help individuals or their friends and families access and monitor their health information. Organizations like Mayo Clinic (2009c) are partnering with these sites to provide users with access to their experts for guidance and support. Others, like Cleveland Clinic (2009), have designed applications to facilitate mass integration of these online patient health records into their system's electronic health record for more effective care coordination.

One study found that approximately 64 percent of U.S. physicians are now downloading apps to PDAs or smart phones to e-prescribe and review laboratory test results. Prescription drug reference is a popular use for this technology and is bolstered by apps for the drug reference program Epocrates, which physicians use to reduce the likelihood of a medication error (Software Advice 2009).

As Exhibit 11.1 illustrates, healthcare smartphone users identified the tasks they would like to see on their phones in the future (Software Advice 2009), which highlights the need for apps that are integrated with the software being used in the facility.

While clinicians use apps to read online journals and medical and drug references (Manhattan Research 2009), some medical schools now require their students to have apps to access digital textbooks and reference materials. When surveyed, 90 percent of

**Exhibit 11.1: Desired Smartphone Functions**

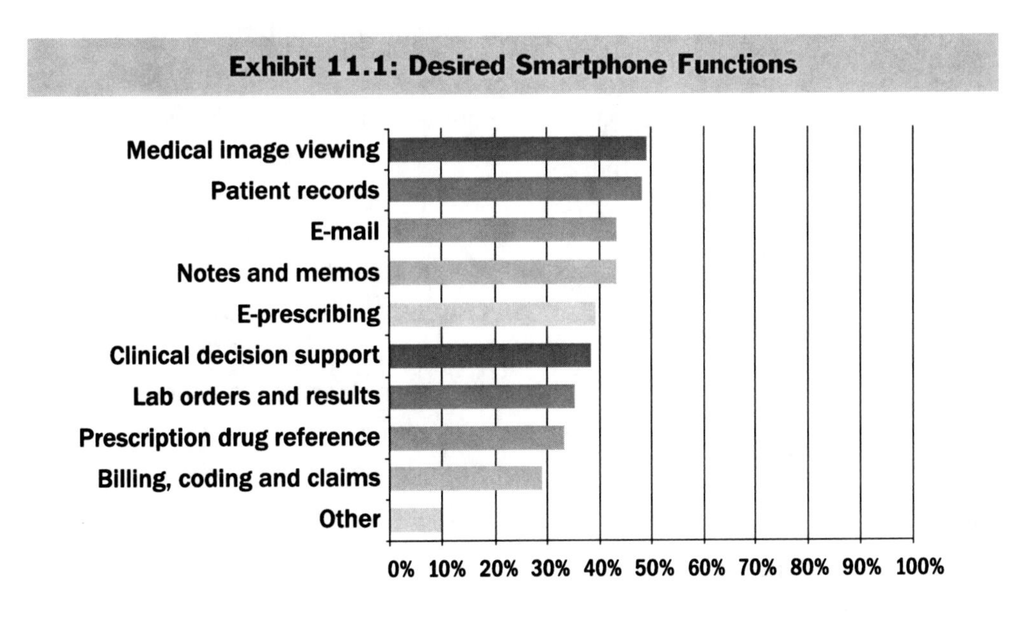


SOURCE: Software Advice (2009). Reprinted with permission.

medical students reported that they view the information available through mobile or online drug and disease references as highly credible, and nearly 60 percent indicated that they use decision-support software at least twice daily to confirm proper drug doses, check for adverse reactions and interactions, and access the disease reference guide (Epocrates 2009). They are also four times more likely to consult a mobile reference for a clinical question than to ask their attending physicians.

### Getting Started

Create a widget of your organization's logo that links back to your website. Place it on your weblog and other social networking sites. Make the code available to partner organizations that can help drive traffic to your site. Widgetbox (www.widgetbox.com) helps organizations create widgets to address specific needs.

Add relevant buttons and badges to your site to enhance its attractiveness and to support other organizations.

Assess the organizational risks related to downloading widgets and applications and making patient information and reference materials accessible on mobile devices. Establish policies and guidelines as appropriate.

## SEARCH ENGINE OPTIMIZATION

**Search engine optimization (SEO)** is an Internet marketing strategy that increases a website's visibility by improving its placement in search results. It aims to have the site show up on the first page of search results. Tactics include managing the content and HTML coding to increase relevance to specific keywords.

---

**Search engine optimization (SEO)**—The process of improving the volume or quality of traffic to a website from search engines via natural (organic or algorithmic) search results. Typically, the earlier a site appears in the search results list, the more visitors it will receive from the search engine. SEO may target different kinds of searches, including image search, local search, and industry-specific vertical search engines.

---

Through keyword analysis, you can determine what words and terms your prospects are searching for.

You can then increase the relevance of your posts by using those same words and terms in your site.

In a U.S. survey, 68 percent of respondents report that they are most likely seeking information on a specific issue or illness when searching for health information online, and 32 percent report that they are seeking information on how to stay well or become healthier. Approximately 44 percent go directly to health-oriented websites, but 35 percent use search engines to find health information. Only 11 percent of respondents have never searched online for health information (Microsoft 2009).

Few commercial Web search engines disclose their search logs, so keyword information is difficult to find. However, Spink and colleagues (2000) analyzed queries from the Excite search engine and found the following:

- The average length of a search query was 2.4 terms.
- About half of the users entered a single query, while almost a third of users entered three or more unique queries.
- Almost half of the users examined only the first one or two pages of results (ten results per page).
- Less than 5 percent of users used advanced search features (e.g., "and," "or," and "not").
- The top three most frequently used terms were "and," "of," and "sex."

Findings from other studies include the following:

- Excite query logs revealed that 19 percent of the queries contained a geographic term (Sanderson and Kohler 2004).
- Yahoo's query logs revealed that 33 percent of the queries from the same user were repeat queries and that 87 percent of the time the user would click on the same result, suggesting that many users use repeat queries to revisit or refind information (Teevan et al. 2006).
- Query term frequency distributions typically conform to the 80/20 rule (20 percent of the terms show up in 80 percent of searches), which allows search engines to employ caching and prefetching (Baeza-Yates 2005).

The healthcare industry as a whole has some work to do in optimizing its online presence and visibility. Stanford University Medical

Center was ranked the sixteenth best hospital in the 2009 *U.S. News & World Report* Best Hospitals list. However, when this same list was evaluated for online presence, One-UpWeb (2009a) ranked Stanford number one—because its search engine ranking on key topics was higher than the rankings of the other hospitals.

As noted in Chapter 2, social media expose your online presence to a wider audience, and as traffic to your website increases, so will its ranking and visibility. In addition to the media described in previous chapters, online publishing platforms such as Blurb (www.blurb.com) and Squidoo (www.squidoo.com) can help increase the online content that links back to your organization's site.

## RSS Feeds

Really Simple Syndication (RSS) feeds send online site (e.g., websites, weblogs, wiki, social networks, etc.) updates to Web-based, desktop, or mobile devices. Those interested in a site can automatically receive any updates to its content, eliminating the need to visit periodically looking for changes. Users subscribe to a feed by entering the URL in a feed reader or clicking on the RSS icon in a browser. The RSS reader monitors the feeds and provides a user interface for the subscriber to receive and read any updates.

RSS feeds are easy to track. And tracking them is important, because these users have actively invited your content into their lives via their e-mail inboxes or an online site. These users could be your most loyal patients, consumers, employees, and the media—people wanting to see what you will come up with next.

## Trackbacks

Trackbacks, which are also known as linkbacks, report links to online pages, posts, or documents. A trackback lets the owner of a page track links to his or her post. They are commonly found in blog posts that reference content in other sites that might interest readers. For example, if a blogger writes a post that references a post on another blog, he or she can include a trackback that allows readers to visit the other blog, rather than repeating what the other blogger wrote. Trackbacks make it easy to create links to your sites on the sites of others and thereby increase traffic. This increased traffic is picked up by the search engines and also contributes to your site's rankings.

### Pings

A ping pushes a weblog link to notify a server that its content has been updated. Blog search engines and aggregators that subscribe to these servers pick up the list of blogs that have recently pinged them and drive traffic to those with the most up-to-date and relevant posts.

### Getting Started

Search engines are the leading tool for attracting consumers who seek online health and wellness information (iCrossing 2008). Optimize your online presence by ensuring that your site includes relevant and indexable content and by following these tips:

- Tag keywords. Know what terms your prospective audience is searching for to ensure that search engines direct these users to your site.
- Submit your site's URL to search engines, site aggregators, and directories.
- Add an RSS button so your readers can subscribe to feeds from your website, blog, or other social networking site.
- Consider ping, trackback, and keyword opportunities for each post.

CHAPTER 12

# Creating a Social Media Plan for Your Health Organization

There is a learning curve for each technology described in this book. If you or your social media team are unfamiliar with the tools, the upfront time investment can be significant. Social media tools should not be taken lightly or applied blindly. The keys to a successful strategy are planning collaboratively and applying the right technology to the right need for the right users.

Social media make up just one piece of your marketing, communications, information, education, or collaboration strategy. Correctly applied, social media tools will build trust and loyalty among stakeholders.

Consumers are driving our use of social media, and some healthcare organizations may find themselves trying to catch up with competitors or watching as e-patients align more closely with other care providers or health plans. The development and implementation of a social media plan increases the ▶

likelihood that your organization will be engaged in the conversation. An effective plan will also help you reach new communities around your region, the nation, and, if you desire, the world.

Physicians, your employees, and your volunteers are already blogging, participating in social networks, or using wikis to collaborate on projects. These individuals represent a pool of collective knowledge and a resource for identifying your strategy, which may include leveraging their existing sites and content to support your brand.

The greatest investment will come from the human assets you already have in your organization rather than any outlay of cash. However, be prepared to expend some resources. These could include the cost of securing a domain name, monthly service fees, or production/equipment costs for videos or podcasts. You should also budget time for staff to contribute to planning activities and setup and maintenance of social media tools.

## PLANNING ACTIVITIES: THE RESEARCH

The planning process should start with an assessment of your readiness for social media. The following questions will help you identify assets and any gaps that will need to be addressed up front.

- What do your executives and informal leaders think about social media?
- What do your employees and physicians think about social media?
- Are there any bloggers in the organization—physicians, employees, board members, volunteers, foundation members?
- Do any of your employees or physicians regularly read blogs or visit social networking sites?
- What social media tools are your physicians, staff, and patients talking about? Using?
- Do you already have content (video, audio) that could be repackaged for use with social media tools?
- Do you already incorporate any social media tools into your website or intranet?
- How many of your employees and physicians carry smartphones or PDAs?

Once you have collected some basic information, conduct a SWOT analysis to identify strengths, weaknesses, opportunities, and threats.

Start by building on your strengths and the online activities of individuals already in your organization. Use their knowledge to help define a strategy that makes sense for your organization. Review best practices in the industry. (The online book companion includes a number of examples.) Identify your organization's communication weaknesses or target populations and establish goals for how you will address those weaknesses and reach out to those groups.

Learn about social media by signing on to LinkedIn, starting a microblog account, or setting up RSS feeds from your favorite websites, social news sites, or blogs. Add widgets like SlideShare to your intranet, and CDC's FluView National Flu Activity Map to your desktop, or add buttons promoting your favorite causes to your organization's website.

As you move through the planning process, take the following actions to further strengthen your plan and, ultimately, its implementation.

- Ensure that your social media strategy includes more than a one-way push of information. Otherwise, your readers will soon realize you don't understand or value connections, multilateral communication, and collaboration.
- Survey your target audiences to find out which social media they are already using. Visit those sites to learn more, and join the conversation once you become comfortable.
- Plan to engage your target audiences in ways that are natural for them and that fit their cultural context.
- Personalize information for the audience and use the technology they prefer.
- Go where the people you want to reach are communicating.
- Determine which technologies are best for your organization, and decide whether the emphasis will be personal or professional.
- Consider the security and privacy needs for each social media tool. Understand that privacy and security considerations are the same whether or not the information is electronic.
- Determine whether a secured or public environment is appropriate.
- Implement controls for connections, friends, and followers.
- Review current policies and procedures and identify areas that need to be revised to accommodate social media technologies.
- Consider how you will manage content and respond to that posted

by readers, particularly when it is negative. Options include the following:
  - Review prior to posting or receive notice whenever a new post is added.
  - Establish ground rules for the community, comment policies, and/or a user agreement.
  - Establish policies and guidelines for employees, medical staff, and others affiliated with your organization.
- Decide who will contribute, review, and approve content and establish clear guidelines. Keep the following suggestions in mind:
  - Ensure that those who participate will have the time to keep information flowing and the content current.
  - Limit the number of individuals who can control the content, but engage everyone involved and your target audience.
- Implement one media tool at a time until you have sufficient support and trust.
- Extend current activities by adding an online component, whenever possible.
- Identify projects to pilot and take advantage of low- or no-cost technologies already available.
- Identify a strategy for Web visibility and measure the positive and negative effects of each tool applied.
- Search for the name of your organization on key sites such as Twitter, MySpace, Facebook, LinkedIn, YouTube, and Wikipedia. Review the content for accuracy and appropriateness and establish a visibility baseline on each site.
- Search for your organization's name and key terms associated with your programs and services using a variety of search engines to learn where your facility's sites rank and establish your SEO baseline.
- Understand what your target audience is searching for and tailor your posts to their interests to establish a solid presence and ensure that they find your site on page one of their search results.
- Secure your organization's name on free social media sites—even those you don't initially plan to use.
- Review your site's content for keywords related to your areas of aggressive growth and specialized or priority service offerings. Consider
  - typical signs and symptoms,
  - targeted diagnosis or conditions, and
  - high-demand "how to" information,

- Review patient satisfaction survey results and suggestion box comments to identify the information your consumers want to find, and consider tagging these terms on your site.
- Work with your webmaster to identify your site's current metatags.
- Determine which of your site's pages receive the most traffic and try to identify the reason. Incorporate your findings into the development of future content.
- Visit Google Analytics (www.google.com/analytics), and consider registering your site to analyze your traffic data and assist with monitoring and reporting.
- Include links to your website on your profile/home pages and in posts on your social media sites.
- Add relevant comments and posts on the sites of others and include linkbacks or trackbacks to your blog or website.
- Select appropriate quantifiable measures of return or value metrics, such as
  - visits to site (traffic),
  - visits by geographic location,
  - number and type of comments to posts,
  - downloads,
  - RSS feeds established,
  - trackbacks, and
  - donations made using the site.
- Maintain a record of more subjective indicators of value or return, and don't disregard the power of sharing the real stories of those affected by your strategy.
- Make it easy to report inappropriate content or to request its removal.

## Suggestions for Specific Media

**Facebook and Twitter** Consider a condition- or disease-specific strategy for Facebook and Twitter, and establish an account or page for each of your key service lines. Healthcare is personal, and this strategy will help your patients connect with those who are most like them and build a tighter and more trusting community.

**Wikipedia** Visit the Contents page of Wikipedia (en.wikipedia.org/wiki/Portal:Contents) to learn more about navigating the site and adding content. If you search for your organization and it is already listed, consider adding or editing the existing content to enhance the presentation.

If your organization is not listed, visit the Wikipedia pages of similar organizations. Use them as examples for creating an article on your facility's history and offerings.

Highlight your centers of excellence or your experts by adding content, research, studies, and reports to appropriate Wikipedia topics. Or add missing topics, subtopics, or content to expand on existing information. This content can include links to reference materials, such as journal articles, research papers, or interviews. Refer to Wikipedia's content criteria (en.wikipedia.org/wiki/Wikipedia:About#Wikipedia_content_criteria) if you have questions about what is acceptable.

**Exhibit 12.1: The PDCA Cycle**

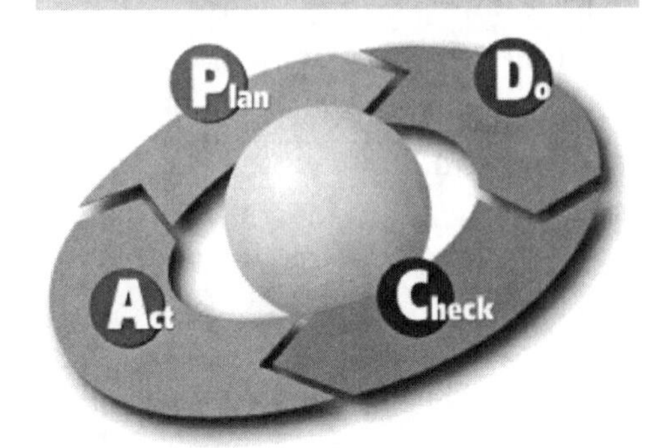


SOURCE: Wikipedia (2009b). Reprinted with permission.

## PREPARING A SOCIAL MEDIA PLAN

Once you are familiar with available social media technologies and how they are currently being used, you are ready to start planning for their application in your organization. Step one is to identify your needs that can be addressed with a social media tool. Turn to the PDCA Cycle (Exhibit 12.1) to help guide you through the planning process for each tool and its application.

### Plan

Establish a project team, and determine your audience and most appropriate form of media and specific tool. Focus on the expected output and establish the objectives and processes necessary to deliver the desired results.

### Do

Implement the new social media tools and processes on a small scale or pilot, if possible.

### Check

Evaluate the new processes. Measure the outcomes and compare your results with the expected results to determine whether any variances exist.

### Act

Analyze the variances to determine cause and identify areas for improvement. If change is necessary, return to the planning phase to refine the audience, form of media, specific tools, expected output, objectives, or process and repeat the remaining steps until you obtain your desired results.

Once you have identified the projects that are most likely to succeed, you are ready to formulate a proposal to present to your colleagues and leaders and begin the broader conversation to initiate your organization's formal social media plan.

CHAPTER 13

# A Vision for the Future

Healthcare is moving away from the idea that the doctor (or hospital) knows best and toward a partnership between clinicians and patients. Consumers are taking more responsibility for expanding their knowledge and making decisions for their own health and wellness. We can expect to see more e-patients and consumers taking an active role in their healthcare education and decisions so that they can

- do as much for themselves and their families as they can,
- ask for the healthcare they and their families need, and
- say no to care they and their families don't need.

The economic downturn is forcing CEOs to take a harder look at the potential benefits of social media tools. At the same time, Web 2.0 solutions are ▶

available to transform operations and organizational cultures. We can expect to see our healthcare CEOs join their peers in other industries by exploring and deploying social media tools to solve communication and collaboration challenges and help their organizations and employees become more effective and efficient.

Healthcare organizations will continue to apply technologies like blogs and wikis to harness the collective wisdom of their staff and broaden collaboration. They will use social media tools to connect with employees, physicians, patients, and other stakeholders and gather the information they need to make more informed decisions. They will avoid missing out on vital information and more quickly identify opportunities to improve performance.

We are transitioning from *unilateral communication* to a new world of *multilateral connections and collaboration*. Mass collaboration will change everything, including how our leaders respond to negative opinions and engage new stakeholders. "To innovate and succeed, the new mass collaboration must become part of every leader's playbook and lexicon. Learning how to engage and cocreate with a shifting set of self-organized partners is becoming an essential skill, as important as budgeting, R&D, and planning" (Tapscott and Williams 2008).

*"To innovate and succeed, the new mass collaboration must become part of every leader's playbook and lexicon. Learning how to engage and cocreate with a shifting set of self-organized partners is becoming an essential skill, as important as budgeting, R&D, and planning."*

We can also expect to see

- our leaders welcome criticism through open conversation;
- a new approach to advertising based on connections and messaging that is "authentic and humble, and built on the principle of a two-way conversation that adds value to the consumer" (Nielsen 2009);
- more movement away from simple broadcast models or "pushed messages" to viral

marketing that leverages powerful networks at little cost and is open to small and large healthcare organizations;

- a transformation in relationships with consumers and more demand for decision-making tools that help them plan and execute what they want;
- the standard practice of medicine incorporate online social media and mobile tools for
  - communicating with patients,
  - educating patients, and
  - monitoring information captured by medical and other devices;
- social media technologies applied to the bedside practice of care and capturing patient data and information in electronic health record systems;
- greater use of mobile devices and applications supporting online networking;
- greater use of social networking sites and an increase in online communities focused on specific segments of the population;
- healthcare leaders working through networks to engage key stakeholders rather than being confined by hierarchies and corporate bureaucracy;
- more online tools to assist consumers with healthcare spending decisions, especially as health system reforms and health savings accounts promote the idea of knowledgeable consumers;
- more people connecting all of their social media using portals, social networking site interaction tools such as Open Social (code.google.com/apis/opensocial), and site aggregators;
- microblogging technology being applied to more and more clinical and operational uses;
- regular use of virtual worlds for orientation, training, and education of staff, patients, and families; and
- greater use of avatars to deliver channels of information missing in other business collaboration tools (Reeves and Read 2009).

Thomas Friedman (2005) concludes his book *The World Is Flat* with a discussion on advances in technology and the need to identify, expose, and capture those who misuse it: "But in the end, technology alone cannot keep us safe. We really do have to find ways to affect the imagination of those who would use the tools of collaboration to destroy the world that has invented those tools."

Advances in social media technology will continue as these tools are more specifically applied in healthcare settings. Healthcare leaders need the knowledge to take full advantage of these tools and to identify, expose, and capture any misuse that threatens the benefits of collaboration.

Hopefully, this book has imparted some new knowledge of social networking and the various media that will keep your healthcare organization on the cutting edge and keep you hip in the eyes of your younger employees and other young people in your life.

# Glossary

A discussion of social media includes terminology that will be unfamiliar to many people, so the definitions of key terms are listed here and in a running glossary throughout the book. Each definition is pulled from Wikipedia (www.wikipedia.com), an online dictionary/encyclopedia that is also an example of one of the tools discussed.

While most of the key words are defined here, there may be others that seem unfamiliar or confusing. Please use your need for a definition or more information as a reason to visit Wikipedia and explore this powerful social networking tool.

**Blog**—(1) A contraction of the term **weblog**; a type of website, usually maintained by an individual with regular entries consisting of commentary, descriptions of events, or other material such as graphics or video. Entries are commonly displayed in reverse-chronological order. (2) To maintain or add content to a blog.

**Health 2.0**—Healthcare characterized by the ability to rapidly share, classify, and summarize individual health information with the goal of improving healthcare systems, experiences, and outcomes. Health 2.0 refers to a number of related concepts including telemedicine, electronic medical records, and the use of the Internet by patients through message boards, blogs, and other systems. A key concept is that patients themselves have greater insight into and control of information generated about them.

**Microblogging**—A form of multimedia blogging that allows users to publish brief text updates or micromedia such as photos or audio clips, either to be viewed by anyone or to be viewed by a restricted group chosen by the user. These messages can be submitted by a variety of means, including text messaging, instant messaging, e-mail, digital audio, or the Web.

**Photo sharing**—Publishing or transferring of a user's digital photos online, enabling the user to share them with others (publicly or privately). Websites and applications that allow the upload and display of images support this function.

**Podcast**—A blend of the words "iPod" and "broadcast." A podcast is a series of digital computer files, usually either audio or video, released periodically and made available for download by means of Web syndication. Like the term "broadcast," "podcast" can refer to the content itself or to the method by which that content is syndicated; the latter is also called *podcasting*. A podcaster is the person who creates the content.

**RSS** (most commonly translated as "really simple syndication")—A family of Web feed formats used to publish frequently updated works—such as blog entries, news headlines, audio, and video—in a standardized format. An RSS document (which is called a "feed," "Web feed," or "channel") includes full or summarized text, plus metadata such as publishing dates and authorship.

**Search engine optimization (SEO)**—The process of improving the volume or quality of traffic to a website from search engines via natural (organic or algorithmic) search results. Typically, the earlier a site appears in the search results list, the more visitors it will receive from the search engine. SEO may target different kinds of searches, including image search, local search, and industry-specific vertical search engines.

**Social bookmarking**—A method for Internet users to store, organize, search, and manage bookmarks of Web pages with the help of metadata, typically in the form of tags.

**Social media**—Online content created by people using highly accessible and scalable publishing technologies. In its most basic sense, social media represents a shift in how people discover, read, and share news, information, and content. It fuses sociology and technology, transforming monologues (a communication from one to many) into dialogues (two-way communication) and democratizes information, transforming content readers into publishers. Social media is popular because it allows people to form online relationships for personal, political, and business use. Businesses also refer to social media as user-generated content (UGC) or consumer-generated media (CGM).

**Social news sites**—Websites that allow users to submit and vote on news stories or other links, thus determining which links are presented. The social news phenomenon has spawned a number of news aggregator sites, which collect and group articles based on Web interest, presenting users with a reflexive news feed.

**Trackback**—One of three types of linkbacks, which are methods for Web authors to request notification when a user links to one of their documents. This enables authors to keep track of who is linking, and so referring, to their articles.

**Video blogging** (sometimes shortened to **vlogging** or **vidblogging**)—A form of blogging for which the medium is video. Entries are regular and often combine embedded video or a video link with supporting text, images, and other metadata. Video logs (vlogs) often take advantage of Web syndication to distribute video over the Internet, using the RSS or Atom syndication formats, for automatic aggregation and playback on mobile devices and personal computers.

**Web 1.0**—A retronym that refers to the state of the World Wide Web and any website design style used before the advent of Web 2.0; a general term created to describe the Web before the bursting of the dot-com bubble in 2001, which was a turning point for the Internet.

**Web 2.0**—A second generation of Web development and Web design. It facilitates communication, information sharing, interoperability, user-centered design, and collaboration on the World Wide Web. It has led to the development and evolution of Web-based communities, hosted services, and Web applications. Examples include social-networking sites, video-sharing sites, wikis, blogs, mashups, and folksonomies.

**Website**—A collection of related Web pages, images, videos, or other digital assets that are addressed with a common domain name or Internet protocol (IP) address in an IP-based network. A website is hosted on at least one Web server, accessible via the Internet or a private local area network.

**Web widget**—A portable chunk of code that can be installed and executed within any separate HTML-based Web page by an end user without requiring additional compilation. Other terms used to describe Web widgets include *gadget, badge, module, webjit, capsule, snippet, mini,* and *flake.* Widgets often take the form of on-screen tools (e.g., clocks, event countdowns, auction tickers, stock market tickers, and flight arrival and daily weather information).

**Wiki**—A website that uses wiki software, allowing users to create and edit any number of interlinked Web pages, using a simplified markup language or a WYSIWYG text editor within the browser. Wikis are often used to create collaborative websites and to power community websites.

# References

AT&T. 2008. "The Business Impacts of Social Networking." [Online document; retrieved 12/2/09.] www.business.att.com/content/whitepaper/WP-soc_17172_v3_11-10-08.pdf.

Baeza-Yates, R. 2005. "Applications of Web Query Mining." [Online article; retrieved 12/21/09.] www.springerlink.com/content/kpphaktugag5mbv0.

Baumann, P. 2009. "Healthcare Is Social." [Online information; retrieved 1/4/10.] www.slideshare.net/philbaumann/140-health-care-uses-for-twitter-presentation.

Beard, L., K. Wilson, D. Morra, and J. Keelan. 2009. "A Survey of Health-Related Activities on Second Life." [Online article; retrieved 12/7/09.] www.jmir.org/2009/2/e17.

Bennet, E. 2009. "Hospital Social Network List." [Online information; retrieved 12/2/09.] ebennett.org/hsnl.

Capps, K. H., and J. B. Barkley, Jr. 2008. "Executive Brief: Employee Health and Wellness and Disease Management Programs." [Online document; retrieved 12/2/09.] www.nam.org/~/media/Files/s_nam/docs/240700/240686.pdf.ashx.

CareerBuilder. 2009. "Forty-Five Percent of Employers Use Social Networking Sites to Research Job Candidates, CareerBuilder Survey Finds." [Online document; retrieved 12/7/09.] www.careerbuilder.com/share/aboutus/pressreleasesdetail.aspx?id=pr519&sd=8%2f19%2f2009&ed=12%2f31%2f2009&siteid=cbpr&sc_cmp1=cb_pr519.

Children's Medical Center. 2009. "From the Red Balloon." [Online information; retrieved 12/3/09.] childrensmedicalcenter.blogspot.com.

Cleveland Clinic. 2009. "Cleveland Clinic Secure Online Services: MyChart." [Online information; retrieved 12/21/09.] my.clevelandclinic.org/eclevelandclinic/mychart/default.aspx.

Cleveland.com. 2009. "Case Western Reserve Univeristy and Second Life Building a Private Virtual World for College." [Online article; retrieved 1/4/10.] www.cleveland.com/education/index.ssf/2009/05/case_western_reserve_universit_5.html.

Coffield, R. 2009. "Health Care Law Blog." [Online information; retrieved 12/2/09.] healthcarebloglaw.blogspot.com.

Compete. 2009. [Online information; retrieved 12/15/09.] siteanalytics.compete.com/digg.com+reddit.com+stumbleupon.com.

Comscore. 2009. "Health Insurance Provider Site Attracts Fewer U.S. Visitors as Unemployment Increases." [Online document; retrieved 12/2/09.] www.comscore.com/layout/set/popup/Press_Events/Press_Releases/2009/8/Health_Insurance_Provider_Sites_Attract_Fewer_U.S._Visitors_as_Unemployment_Increases.

eMarketer. 2009. "Podcasting: Into the Mainstream." [Online information; retrieved 12/8/09.] www.emarketer.com/Report.aspx?code=emarketer_20000569.

Epocrates. 2009. "Future Physicians Weigh in on Importance of Technology in Medicine." [Online article; retrieved 12/21/09.] www.epocrates.com/company/news/082009.html.

Ferguson, T. 2007. "E-Patients: How They Can Help Us Heal Healthcare." [Online document; retrieved 12/1/09.] www.e-patients.net/e-Patients_White_Paper.pdf.

Fox, S., and S. Jones. 2009. "The Social Life of Health Information." [Online document; retrieved 12/2/09.] www.pewinternet.org/Reports/2009/8-The-Social-Life-of-Health-Information.aspx.

Friedman, T. L. 2005. *The World Is Flat: A Brief History of the Twenty-First Century*. New York: Farrar, Straus and Giroux.

Harrington, B. 2009. "iCrossing POV: Twitter." [Online document; retrieved 12/3/09.] www.icrossing.com/articles/iCrossing-Twitter-101-April-09.pdf.

iCrossing. 2008. "How America Searches: Health and Wellness." [Online document; retrieved 12/2/09.] www.icrossing.com/research/how-america-searches-health-and-wellness.php.

Jain, S. H. 2009. "Practicing Medicine in the Age of Facebook." *New England Journal of Medicine* 361 (7): 649–51.

Kemper, D. W., and M. Mettler. 2008. "E-Coaching for Boomer Health." [Online document; retrieved 12/2/09.] hwinfo.healthwise.org/docs/DOCUMENT/8248.pdf.

Langshur, S. 2008. "Online Care Gets Personal." [Online document; retrieved 12/2/09.] cms.carepages.com/export/sites/default/CarePages/en/Press/white_papers/online_health_care_gets_personal.pdf.

Lemley, T., and J. F. Burnham. 2008. "Web 2.0 Tools in Medical and Nursing School Curricula." *Journal of the Medical Library Association* 97 (1): 50–52.

Manhattan Research. 2009. *Taking the Pulse v9.0*. New York: Manhattan Research.

Mathews, A. W. 2009. "Health Insurers Eye Social Networking." [Online information; retrieved 12/2/09.] blogs.wsj.com/health/2009/08/19/health-insurers-eye-social-networking.

Mayo Clinic. 2009a. "Blog Comment Policy." [Online information; retrieved 12/3/09.] www.mayoclinic.org/blogs/comment.html.

Mayo Clinic. 2009b. "For Mayo Clinic Employees." [Online information; retrieved 12/3/09.] sharing.mayoclinic.org/guidelines/for-mayo-clinic-employees.

Mayo Clinic. 2009c. "Mayo Clinic Health Manager." [Online information; retrieved 12/21/09.] healthmanager.mayoclinic.com/default.aspx.

Microsoft. 2009. "Health Engagement Survey." [Online information; retrieved 12/21/09.] www.microsoft.com/downloads/details.aspx?FamilyID = B67655EA-F60A-4E55-93B4-6B5ABF6347F7&displaylang = en.

Nielsen. 2009a. "Global Faces and Networked Places: A Nielsen Report on Social Networking's New Global Footprint." [Online document; retrieved 12/2/09.] blog.nielsen.com/nielsenwire/wp-content/uploads/2009/03/nielsen_globalfaces_mar09.pdf.

Nielsen. 2009b. "Nielsen's Social Media QuickTake: May 2009."[Online document; retrieved 12/3/09.] www.blog.nielsen.com/nielsenwire/wp-content/uploads/2009/06/nielsen_pr_090619.pdf.

Noblis. 2007. "*HotZone*: First Responder Game." [Online document; retrieved 12/7/09.] noblis.com/MethodsTools/AreasofExpertise/Documents/HotZone.pdf.

OneUpWeb. 2009a. "America's Hospitals and Online Marketing: Do They Get It?" [Online article; retrieved 12/21/09.] www.oneupweb.com/white-papers/americas_hospit.

———. 2009b. "The Fusion of Search and Social Media." [Online document; retrieved 12/2/09.] www.oneupweb.com/library/whitepapers.

———. 2006. "The Power and Principles of Podcasting. A Comprehensive Guide to Corporate Podcasting." [Online document; retrieved 12/8/09.] www.oneupweb.com/library/whitepapers.

Pronin, E., and D. Wegner. 2008. "Manic Thinking: Independent Effects of Thought Speed and Thought Content on Mood." *Psychological Science* 17 (9): 807–13.

Reeves, B., and J. L. Read. 2009. *Total Engagement: Using Games and Virtual Worlds to Change the Way People Work and Businesses Compete.* Boston: Harvard Business Press.

Sanderson, M., and J. Koehler. 2004. "Analyzing Geographic Queries." [Online article; retrieved 12/21/09.] www.geo.unizh.ch/~rsp/gir/abstracts/sanderson.pdf.

Software Advice. 2009. "Survey Results: Which Smartphone Will Own the Healthcare Market?" [Online information; retrieved 12/21/09.] www.softwareadvice.com/articles/ medical/smartphone-survey-results-1073009.

Socialtext. 2009. "Five Best Practices for Enterprise Collaboration Success." [Online document; retrieved 12/1/09.] www.socialtext.com/offers/wp_bestpractices_readwriteweb.php.

Spink, A., D. Wolfram, B. J. Janson, and T. Saracevic. 2000. "Searching the Web: The Public and Their Queries." *Journal of the American Society for Science and Technology* 52 (3): 226–34.

Stanford University School of Medicine, Center for Immersive and Simulation-Based Learning. 2009. "Desktop Simulations and Virtual Worlds." [Online information; retrieved 12/7/09.] cisl.stanford.edu/what_is/sim_modalities/desktop_sim.html.

Tapscott, D., and A. Williams. 2008. *Wikinomics: How Mass Collaboration Changes Everything.* New York: Portfolio.

Teevan, J., E. Adar, R. Jones, and M. Potts. 2006. "History Repeats Itself: Repeat Queries in Yahoo's Logs." [Online article; retrieved 12/21/09.] people.csail.mit.edu/teevan/work/publications/posters/sigir06.pdf.

Thielst, C. B. 2007. "Weblogs: A Communication Tool." *Journal of Healthcare Management* 52 (5): 287–89.

U.S. Bank. 2008. "Health Savings Solution." [Online information; retrieved 12/2/09.] www.healthsavings.usbank.com/.

VizEdu. 2009. "Twitter and Health 2.0." [Online document; retrieved 12/3/09.] vizedu.com/2009/01/twitter-and-health-20/.

Wellsphere. 2009. "BeWell@Stanford." [Online information; retrieved 12/7/09.] stanford.wellsphere.com/home.s.

Wikipedia. 2009a. "GUI Widget." [Online articles; retrieved 12/17/09.] en.wikipedia.org/ wiki/GUI_widget.

Wikipedia. 2009b. "PDCA." [Online article; retrieved 12/23/09.] en.wikipedia.org/wiki/PDCA.

Wikipedia. 2009c. "Wikipedia: About." [Online article; retrieved 12/14/09.] en.wikipedia.org/wiki/Wikipedia:About.

# Acknowledgments

To Doc Searls, who opened my eyes to the possibilities of blogs, wikis, and pinging. (http://blogs.law.harvard.edu/doc/)

To Phil Baumann; Kelly Leslie Hall; Lisa Wehr; Maureen Mallory; Chuck Dorman; Charles Quesenberry; Ed Bennett; Marty Bonick; Terry Behunin; Michal Sandoff; Kristine Olsen; Gale Wilson Steele; Laurie Schueler; Ron Jimenez, MD; Judith Smith; Robert Coffield; Maureen Michaels; Dennis Kotecki; Mary Margaret Crulcich; Edward Prentice III; Martin Harris, MD; Lee Aase; Geoff Rutledge, MD; and Jessica Newell, who so graciously helped me identify and share our social media best practices.

To my supportive and ever-loving family who allow me to follow my professional passions—Geoff, Catherine, Christian, and Sarah!

# About the Author

Christina Beach Thielst is an administrator with a long career in a variety of hospital and other healthcare settings who has experienced firsthand the challenges and barriers to effective communications and collaboration. She sees great potential for correctly applied social media tools in healthcare environments.

In July 2005, she started her weblog, Christina's Considerations (thielst .typepad.com), in an effort to collect, organize, and share digital information related to her professional interest and work. Her blog has helped her find and use her voice on current healthcare issues, and she continually incorporates new social media tools and technologies. Today, she has not only a Web presence, but also Web visibility.

Christina has a master's in health administration from Tulane University School of Public Health and Tropical Medicine and is a fellow of the American College of Healthcare Executives. She is on the board of Healthcare Executives of Southern California and is a member of the Health Information Management Systems Society.

Her first book, *Guide to Establishing a Regional Health Information Exchange*, was published by HIMSS in 2007.

Have a question or comment for Christina? Visit her weblog at thielst .typepad.com or send Christina a tweet at Twitter:@Cthielst. You can also visit her LinkedIn page at www.linkedin.com/in/christinathielst.